LAURETTE WILLIS REAC

"Laurette realizes every busy woman has a need to be fit in body, soul, and spirit. In *The Busy Woman's Guide to Total Fitness,* under 'Your Fitness Personality,' she shows how The Personalities help point the way to discovering a fitness plan best suited for each personality type. Amazing what can be accomplished in only 20 minutes a day!"

FLORENCE LITTAUER
Founder, The CLASS Seminar,
speaker, author of *Personality Plus* and *Silver Boxes*

"We encourage our clients and patients to exercise on a regular basis and find the PraiseMoves program to be a complement to our practice!"

DR. AMY C. DENMAN, CTN
Alternative Chiropractic

"I am so thankful to have PraiseMoves, the Christian alternative to yoga that leads participants into deeper relationship with the Lord."

THERESA STAHL, RD, LDN

"Through regular use of PraiseMoves I have regained the flexibility and energy I thought was gone forever. The best part: I continue to grow in wisdom and knowledge of our wonderful Lord and Savior, Jesus Christ!"

Julie Wood

"Since doing PraiseMoves I notice I no longer have PMS symptoms or migraine headaches. They're gone!"

Stephanie Cavnar

"I come away from PraiseMoves feeling closer to the Lord and have a stronger body, more flexibility, better circulation...Laurette Willis quotes scripture during the exercise time and that really helps me hide God's Word in my heart. To exercise spiritually and physically is really a blessing!"

L. Gordoni

"PraiseMoves is a wonderful treat for my body; it is effective yet gentle (just what my spirit and my stressed-out, middle-aged body needs!)."

Linda Kleidon

"Laurette Willis has a very unique gifting in her ability to portray great women of the Bible. She 'became' Mary Magdalene and Priscilla. We were transported back in time! Laurette's attention to the details added to the authenticity. She is a talented actress and exceptionally used by God to present the message of salvation.

"Laurette also presented her exceptional workshop 'Fitness for His Witness.' This was a huge success."

ELEANOR GROSSGLASS
Women's Ministry director,
New York District Council of the Assemblies of God

"The children and staff enjoyed your program. I was amazed at how well you captivated a group of 2nd and 3rd graders. The themes you used, such as deception and honesty, go along with our character education program. The best thing is students learned about history, storytelling, acting, and character building in an innovative and fun way."

JANET RICHARDSON
Counselor, William R. Teague Elementary

"It was our pleasure to have Laurette Willis come to our church for a wonderful weekend of laughter, entertainment, and anointed ministry. She brought the house down as she performed songs, imitated famous voices and sound effects, and used audience interaction. On Sunday morning she performed 'Mary Magdalene' from her one-woman show *Great Women of the Bible*. The Bible stories came alive!"

MICKEY KEITH
senior pastor, Life Community Church, and
president, Independent Assemblies Fellowship
of Churches and Ministries

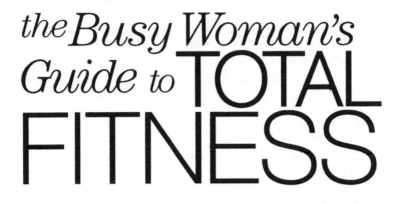

the Busy Woman's Guide to TOTAL FITNESS

Laurette Willis
Author of *Basic Steps to Godly Fitness*

HARVEST HOUSE PUBLISHERS

EUGENE, OREGON

Cover photo © Andrejs Pidjass / iStockphoto

Interior photos © Mike Brown

Cover by Koechel Peterson & Associates, Inc., Minneapolis, Minnesota

THE BUSY WOMAN'S GUIDE TO TOTAL FITNESS
Copyright © 2007 by Laurette Willis
Published by Harvest House Publishers
Eugene, Oregon 97402
www.harvesthousepublishers.com

Library of Congress Cataloging-in-Publication Data

Willis, Laurette,
The busy woman's guide to total fitness / Laurette Willis.
  p. cm.
  ISBN-13: 978-0-7369-1995-1 (pbk.)
  ISBN-10: 0-7369-1995-3 (pbk.)
  1. Physical fitness for women. 2. Physical fitness for women—Psychological aspects. 3. Exercise for women. 4. Spiritual exercises. I. Title.
  GV482.W55 2007
  613.7′045—dc22

                                                    2007020553

Printed in the United States of America

07 08 09 10 11 12 13 14 15 / VP-SK / 11 10 9 8 7 6 5 4 3 2 1

To all the women who have said, "I'm too busy to exercise" or "Eating healthy is too hard to figure out; it takes too much time!" or "Where do I start? Help!" I've been there. I pray this book will be a blessing to you and will help you get fit faster with energy to spare and that you feel better as a result!

To women in Christian ministry: missionaries, teachers, pastors, evangelists, prophets, encouragers, givers and exhorters, prayer warriors, praise and worship leaders, choir members; pastors' wives, women's ministry directors and cell-group leaders; nursery workers, kitchen and cleaning crews, transportation providers, and short-term mission workers, as well as all those in the multifaceted help ministries—plus mothers, daughters, grandmothers, sisters, and aunts who care for children, the elderly, or the infirm. To every woman whose work or service falls under the "as to the Lord" category in Colossians 3:23 ("Whatever you do, do it heartily, as to the Lord and not to men").

To all of us who want to experience God's best and be all He has created us to be.

Contents

WE'RE ALL BUSY

Many shall run to and fro,
and knowledge shall increase.

DANIEL 12:4

Once upon a time the customary reply to the question "How are you doing?" was "Fine, thank you. And you?" Today the answer is "Busy!" Is that you? Do you sometimes feel burdened keeping up with the schedules of everyone in your household? If you're single, do the demands of work and life feel overwhelming at times? Do you feel as if there aren't enough hours in the day to get everything done? Are you finding it difficult to make daily quiet time with the Lord a priority? Is it a challenge to find time to relax, let alone squeeze fitness into your day?

Then you're a busy woman, and this book is for you! There are simple ways you can incorporate health and fitness for spirit, soul, and body into your day and actually have *more* time and energy to do all you're called to do.

Hectic schedules seldom leave time for two very important parts of a well-balanced life: nurturing our relationship with God and keeping our bodies strong and healthy. Since our schedules probably won't be overflowing with extra time in the near future, we must discover ways to make the best use of the time we do have. One way is blending the spiritual and the physical for "Total Fitness."

God is interested in our schedules. Before I made time with the Lord a daily priority, I wondered why I never seemed to have enough time for everything I needed to do. I didn't realize that every area of my life was suffering because I didn't have my priorities in the right order. I needed to give God first place in my life and seek Him above all else.[1] When I began investing time in my relationship with the Lord every morning, I found the peace and wisdom to handle what came my way the rest of the day.

We don't often think of fitness as one of our top life priorities until we experience a health challenge. Then suddenly our physical well-being becomes very important. Have you ever considered that your physical fitness (or lack of it) is important to God, too? I see it this way: I want to go to heaven, but I certainly don't want to go there before my time. We all want the Lord to look at us and say, "Well done, good and faithful servant."[2] No one wants to hear, "Well, what are you doing here so soon?"

The Lord delights in being part of everything we do—even exercise! One woman I know respectfully calls Him her Personal Trainer. When we ask the Lord to be with us during workouts, physical activity is no longer drudgery but an extension of our worship time with Him. His joy—the joy of the Lord—lifts and strengthens us spiritually and emotionally. Building physical strength at the same time becomes an added bonus. Instead of dreading the coming workout, brisk walk, or whatever our fitness routine entails, we'll look forward to being in His presence again.

I've Been Down That Trail Before!

Let's look at the title of this book again: *The Busy Woman's Guide to Total Fitness.* We've already agreed that you qualify for busy, right? So let's consider what a guide to total fitness is. A guide can be a handbook of information or instruction as well as a person who shows the way. The only guidebook worth reading is an accurate one, and the only guide worth following is someone who's traveled the path we're taking. We certainly don't want to follow an outdated map or a guide who hasn't been along the trail before.

I've not only been down the total fitness trail before; I've worn deep ruts along side roads leading to diet dead ends and fitness failure. Those familiar with my book *BASIC Steps to Godly Fitness* (Harvest House, 2005) will recall my 30-year arm-wrestling tournament with food (wrestling to keep food out of my mouth and in my mouth at the same time). My first realization that I had a problem with food came at the age of six. All food was comfort food I used for a variety of reasons: to stave off boredom, to provide entertainment, to be a "friend" to a lonely little girl, to act as a survival tool to numb emotional pain and fill an aching void on the inside that I couldn't explain.

After years of involvement in metaphysics, yoga, and New Age religion (aka "looking for God in all the wrong places"), I surrendered my life to Jesus Christ in 1987. Although I felt profound peace and joy for the first time in my life, not all of my problems disappeared overnight. But a few of them did! The Lord miraculously delivered me from alcoholism—without my even asking Him to do so! His mercy lifted me out of the darkness of feeling compelled to drink wine almost every day and often becoming drunk. On that glorious day, April 1, 1987, the desire to drink alcohol left me—it's completely gone! Then four days after my salvation experience, I met my precious husband, Paul. My loneliness was completely gone! The need for cigarettes, worldly distractions, and mind-numbing entertainment soon left as well.

If only the food issues in my life had been so miraculously removed.

Have you heard the expression, "The Lord will only allow you to experience what you can bear?" It seems to be a variation of 1 Corinthians 10:13:

> No temptation has overtaken you except such as is common to man; but God is faithful, who will not allow you to be

tempted beyond what you are able, but with the temptation will also make the way of escape, that you may be
able to bear it.

Like many women, I found that food, exercise, and body image
were the areas where I faced the greatest temptation, humiliation,
defeat, and guilt. *Lord, help me!* I'd cry. I remember falling to my
knees, my hand on the refrigerator door, praying for God to remove
the temptation to overeat. This happened again and again.

What a loser! a voice in my head taunted.

"Oh, what's the use?" I'd whimper as I pulled open the refrigerator door to stuff my face with "comfort" food. If I truly knew the
Comforter, why was I still giving way to my addiction to this fake
comfort? Oh, the guilt.

Even though the Lord miraculously removed my 13-year addiction to alcohol, and I was able to conquer a 20-year addiction to
nicotine through prayer and fasting, overcoming emotional eating
was a different challenge.

Finally a 12-step recovery program[3] was one of the tools the Lord
led me to and used to help me let go of the emotional baggage that
caused me to use food for reasons other than physical sustenance.
The support and acceptance I received from that group enabled me
to come to terms with why I continued to sabotage every diet and
fitness program I'd tried since I was 11 years old.

Victory in this area is still a daily walk for me that requires honest
self-examination and living out the apostle Paul's admonition to the
Galatians: "Stand fast therefore in the liberty by which Christ has
made us free, and do not be entangled again with a yoke of bondage."[4] Unlike alcohol and cigarettes that are no longer part of my
life, food still is, by necessity, so it's important I remain watchful
and vigilant. I choose not to fool myself by thinking I can go on a
weekend binge and get back on track Monday morning. The Lord
has been so gracious to me in this area that it's important for me to
"stand fast" and hold my ground one day at a time in this glorious
freedom in Him.

Not everyone needs the help of a support group outside the church. Maybe you have friends that provide the support you need through prayer and fellowship. However, for those who need additional help, there are now Christ-centered recovery programs available. Celebrate Recovery is one of these groups.[5] There may even be a meeting at a church near you.

Fitness Can Be Balanced

I was relieved to find among the definitions for "fitness" the words "proper, right, healthy, and balanced." Balance sounds doable—as if we're halfway there already! Achieving total fitness will involve a focused, Spirit-led decision on your part to be healthy in spirit, soul, and body. Notice that the spiritual part of you—where you're already perfect in Christ!—takes preeminence.

My prayer is that this book will serve as a guidebook for you and that I will be a fit guide (in more ways than one!) as you embark on your Total Fitness journey.

FITNESS FOR THE SPIRIT, SOUL, AND BODY = TOTAL FITNESS

Beloved, I wish above all things that thou mayest prosper and be in health, even as thy soul prospereth.

3 JOHN 2 KJV

"Total Fitness" is fitness for the whole person—spirit, soul, and body. You are a spirit. You have a soul (your mind, will, and emotions), and you live in a body (your earth suit). You may not always think of your spirit as the *real* you, but since you are made in the image of God, and God is Spirit, your spirit *is* the real you.

To improve fitness and health in the long run, it's important that you find solutions not only for improving your physical health but for nurturing your emotional and spiritual well-being, too. It all works together. Besides, busy women don't have time to waste on programs that address only part of the problem. Why go just part of the way? Let's take the Total Fitness journey together—with the Lord.

The Total Fitness Journey

By seeing Total Fitness as a journey we're taking together with the Lord rather than as a destination we're trying to reach on our own, we can experience spiritual and emotional progress while improving our physical fitness. That was the problem with all the diets I'd been on before. I only measured the physical changes I experienced. I was trying to reach a special number on the scale or on a clothing tag instead of gauging my true success by the changes that were taking place on the inside.

If there's no change on the inside (in mind, will, and emotion), all the physical changes in the world won't matter. No wonder I continued to sabotage myself whenever I made positive steps toward change. Physical changes alone were never enough. I continued to act and feel like the "same old, same old," so I persisted in the same old behavior. As an unhappy, unfulfilled person who didn't know how to yield to the Holy Spirit and the fruit He brings of faithfulness, patience, and self-control, I didn't have a healthy relationship with food and exercise (Galatians 5:22-23). I saw my diet and fitness regimen as a jail term I was obligated to fulfill. Once the sentence was served, I went back to the old way of doing things because the person on the inside hadn't changed.

I wasn't alone. Some sources say that 8 out of 10 people who go on diets will regain any weight lost; others say that only 5 percent of dieters manage to keep the weight off for more than 5 years. That's a 95 percent failure rate! Something's wrong with that picture. Part of the problem is that most diet and exercise programs focus on motivating us to make physical changes in our lives through the power of our wills. Very few incorporate the use of Scripture and *Holy Spirit* power to bring about *real* change in our body *and* soul.

Transformation in the way we think, respond, and see ourselves will enable us to maintain a healthy lifestyle. We won't want to go back to the old ways because we think differently and see ourselves in a new light.

A Move of God

Do you remember how you felt when you first turned your life over to the Lord? (If you aren't a Christian but would like to know more about what it means, see the "Special Invitation" section at the end of this book.) Even if you came to Christ as a small child, you've probably renewed your commitment as an adult. The Lord provides us with many opportunities to give more of ourselves to Him in our lives. I call these places "surrendering at a deeper depth."

When you make a decision to live your life differently, some pursuits no longer interest you. Certain television shows, magazines, or novels that used to fill your time are no longer appealing. Gossip and backbiting are no longer sports you want to engage in. Sometimes this shift happens instantaneously when you embark on your new commitment to the Lord. You seem to be carried to a new place in the Spirit or you're given a spiritual push in the right direction. You begin to see things through new eyes. Your spiritual senses are sharpened, and you have a new appreciation for what it means to walk in the Spirit. Some old desires are gone and replaced by new desires. Willpower didn't change them; it was an inside job. You could say your "want to" had suddenly changed.

When the Lord in His mercy delivered me from alcoholism the moment I surrendered my life to Him, and the desire to drink alcohol left me completely, I didn't want to hang out in bars (even the fancy ones!). I no longer chose restaurants based on whether they had a wine list. Such thoughts didn't even enter my mind anymore. It was a miraculous transformation and a perfect example of God's mercy at work in a new believer's life.

Do you believe you can make a focused, Spirit-led decision about your health and fitness and receive immediate help from the Lord? Can you experience an overnight change in an area of your life that would cause you to put on your "Hallelujah Jumping Shoes" and have a praise party? Certainly! God specializes in "suddenly" moments.

And Suddenly...

Are there problems in your life that you've been praying about for years? Have you tried in your own power to make changes happen, but to no avail? You *can* trust God to move in those areas of your life. He may bring about change gradually over time, or He may move suddenly and dramatically. The Bible describes a number of instances when people prayed and waited on the Lord—and suddenly things changed. In Acts 16, Paul and Silas were in prison, badly beaten and in chains because of their faith in Jesus. Instead of moaning, wailing, and complaining, they sang praises loud enough that the other prisoners heard them:

> At midnight Paul and Silas were praying and singing hymns to God, and the prisoners were listening to them. *Suddenly* there was a great earthquake, so that the foundations of the prison were shaken; and *immediately* all the doors were opened and everyone's chains were loosed.[1]

See those words "suddenly" and "immediately"? There was a *sudden* earthquake, which not only set Paul and Silas free but released the other prisoners from their chains as well. They wouldn't have experienced freedom, however, if they hadn't been willing to stand up and walk out of their prison cells. They had to start walking! I imagine it must have felt strange at first, especially for those who had been locked in their cells a long time. Some may have been bound by shackles fastened to the walls of the jail. They had to become willing to relearn some things and take more personal responsibility than they had been. They could no longer lean on the old excuses, such as "I can't do that because I'm stuck in this prison. Besides, even though I'm in prison, it's a predictable existence. I feel secure here."

I can relate to that. For years I felt trapped in the prison of my body. I hated the way I looked and felt, and I allowed those feelings to dictate my actions. I didn't go to dinner parties or out with friends. I certainly didn't go swimming with anyone because of how horrible I thought I looked in a swimsuit. I remember feigning sickness when I was 12 years old just to keep from having to go to a pool party! My prison was on the inside, and the lack of freedom gave me a warped sense of security, a place where I felt safe.

Since I surrendered my life to the Lord He has helped me learn to walk as a free woman one day at a time. There are times when the desire to follow the old way of doing things arises. I then have the choice to either pass the test by leaning on the Lord and walking in freedom with Him or retreat to the prison existence. If I choose the latter, I won't go much further in my walk with the Lord until I face the challenge and ask Him to help me overcome it. It's my choice. Walking in freedom is optional.

No diet or exercise program can tear down the prison walls on the inside of us. If we still see ourselves as prisoners to the past and our old behaviors, reaching the perfect weight or size won't make the difference we thought or hoped it would.

I remember going on a water fast when I was 20 years old. It was for purely selfish reasons; there was nothing spiritual about it. I wanted to get skinny fast! I lost so much weight I looked sick, but I still felt fat. When I started eating again, I went back to my old habits and quickly regained the weight I'd lost—with an extra 10 pounds for good measure. I hadn't lost the weight of the burden I was carrying on the inside—the weight of the emotional chains that bound me. That was my true prison.

By the amazing grace of God I've experienced several wonderful "suddenly" deliverances. Other prisons inside me have been torn down one brick at a time, one step at a time. When we experience victory in one area of our lives, it's important that we remain alert and "stand fast" in our new liberty in Christ, giving no ground to the enemy by entertaining old thought patterns and behaviors. This way we'll keep from becoming "entangled again with a yoke of bondage."[2]

One Day at a Time

While "suddenly" moments are wonderful, we seldom know when they're going to happen so most changes happen gradually. These learning experiences take place over time as changes we walk out by faith. After committing your life to the Lord, you may have noticed that as you devoted time to reading the Bible and learning about how God wants you to live your life, you began making different choices. Perhaps you stopped relying on your own power to change people and situations and began bringing your concerns to the Lord. Did you find that situations and relationships began to change the more you surrendered them to Him?

You can experience the same thing in your Total Fitness journey. The more you make healthful decisions in diet (choosing more unprocessed, nutrient-dense foods and saner portions) and exercise (pursuing a more active lifestyle instead of making exercise a dreaded duty), the more these new habits will become part of who you are.

Another way gradual change occurs is during our daily walk with the Lord. You may sense from time to time what some call a "check" in your spirit, a gentle nudge (or sometimes not so gentle!) that lets you know you need to do something differently. That's an example of the wonderful guidance of the Holy Spirit within you. Following His prompting directs, protects, and transforms you.

These examples of spirit and soul change—instantaneous and gradual—shape the way we see ourselves. Our desires change, prompting us to dwell on different thoughts, which leads to more positive, life-affirming actions.

Can you see a parallel here between what can happen on a spiritual level and how similar experiences can affect you emotionally and physically? Some changes may be swift and sudden, while others may happen gradually. Either way, God is faithful, and His promises to you in His Word are true.

In upcoming chapters, you'll learn how to bring about positive physical changes in your life. And you'll also discover ways to apply the Word of God personally, pray for loved ones, and overcome the challenges you face in every area of your life—physical, emotional, and spiritual.

Nothing by Osmosis

After a while I discovered that diets and exercise routines could only do so much for me, and they did *nothing* by osmosis (effortless absorption). The books and videos I bought had little effect on me as long as they sat unheeded on my bookshelf. I had to follow their advice to experience results.

Oh, the thrill I had when I purchased a new book or DVD! "Yea, I did it!" I'd cheer. "Watch out world, here I come!" I felt excitement because I associated crossing the finish line with the purchase of the product. But buying running shoes for the race isn't the same as running or winning the race!

When I brought a book home, I'd leaf through the pages and perhaps even follow the dietary advice for a few days. I'd take a DVD out of the box and watch it a time or two. I always ended up wondering what went wrong. Why couldn't I stick to a plan for more than a few days? Have you ever experienced something similar? Many people don't seem to be able to stick to a new fitness regimen for more than a few days or weeks. Why is that?

The answer is in our "want to"! The change that needs to take place is in our souls—our minds, wills, and emotions. It's an inside job. Our "want to" has to change for us to stick with any new diet or exercise program. And for our desires to change, we need to experience a serious overhaul in the way we see ourselves. As long as I saw myself as someone who failed, who was overweight, who was unmotivated to exercise, who was always uncomfortable with myself, guess what? My experiences became self-fulfilling prophecies and reflections of how I saw myself.

I remember times when a diet was working (aka I was working the diet!). It scared me a little. Yes, I was excited to see positive changes. I liked seeing my tummy become flatter, but deep inside I couldn't really believe it would last. Why? I still saw myself as someone who couldn't be successful. I didn't see myself as a healthy, fit person. I had a poor self-image that wasn't tied to the Word of God and how God made me.

Some might say that my image of God wasn't that big, either. Often it's not how we esteem ourselves but how we esteem God that matters. If we don't really think He cares about the things that concern us, it's difficult to trust that He will help us reach our goals or sustain us when we're weak.

How the Lord Sees You

Scripture reminds us that the Lord is touched by our feelings and infirmities. Jesus was "tempted in every way just as we are—yet was without sin."[3] You are precious to the Lord, made in His own image. Father God has your every tear saved in a little bottle in heaven, and you are inscribed on the palm of His hand.[4] He is "the LORD who heals you."[5] He made you. You are completely "accepted in the Beloved"[6] just as you are. God wants to help you be the best you can possibly be in every area of life.

While our heavenly Father loves us just as we are, He also loves us too much to leave us as we are. He is calling us up higher in our relationship with Him. Isn't that wonderful?

How *does* God see you? The best way to know for sure and to change how you think about yourself is to realize that since you surrendered your life to Jesus Christ, God the Father sees you "in Christ."[7] As you read your New Testament, underline or highlight all of the "in Him," "in Christ," "in whom," and "through Him" scriptures you find. There are approximately 140 of these expressions, most of them in the Epistles (letters Paul and the other apostles wrote to the New Testament churches). When you find one of these "in Christ" scriptures, stop and meditate on it. The Word (Jesus) is speaking about you! Write these scriptures down in your journal or on index cards that you can keep in your Bible or purse or put in different places around the house where you'll see them often. Confess these scriptures aloud, claiming them for yourself: "This is who God says I am because I am in Christ!" The mirror of the Word is the most accurate mirror you can use. Speak the truth of God's Word over yourself and your loved ones instead of repeating what the world and the enemy say out of doubt and unbelief.

When our self-esteem is tied to God's esteem for us, it's possible to believe Him and His Word for big, seemingly impossible things (as long as they line up with what the Bible says is His will for us). We've already discovered that prosperity and being in good health qualify as some of the good things the Lord desires for us to have. No matter what your personal experiences may be, God wants to help you, and His will for you is always good.

It doesn't seem coincidental that health and prosperity in God's eyes are tied to the development of our souls. When we put the Lord first and become willing to see ourselves as He sees us (through fellowship with Him, prayer, meditation on and confession of His Word), our souls will prosper. Our minds, wills, and emotions will thrive and be strengthened to the point where it will become easier to yield to the Holy Spirit and His fruit in our lives, an essential part of a disciplined lifestyle. (I call this "yielding to the fruit of the Spirit," which we'll discuss in more depth later in this chapter.)

Suddenly we're not alone on this journey! The Lord is working changes *in* us, *with* us, and *through* us. We can commit our way to Him and know that He will direct our thoughts and guide and order our steps.[8] We can then yield to His direction and have long-lasting results in every area of our lives.

If You Know How to Worry, You Know How to Meditate

The Bible gives us the perfect prescription for change: "Don't copy the behavior and customs of this world, but let God transform you into a new person by changing the way you think. Then you will learn to know God's will for you, which is good and pleasing and perfect."[9]

We're to *let* God transform us. You and I are part of this process. Meditate on the Word of God and let Him change the way you think. How do you meditate? If you know how to worry, you know how to meditate. I learned a long time ago that worrying is little more than meditating on what the devil wants to see happen in our lives. We've all worried, and since the Bible says that "whatever is not from faith is sin,"[10] worry certainly qualifies, doesn't it? So let's turn to the Lord in faith whenever we're tempted to worry and meditate on His Word instead.

How is worrying like meditation? Think of it this way: Just as you can go over and over a worrisome thought or scenario, you can take a portion of Scripture and go over it in your mind, considering every angle. Speak the Scripture aloud, then dwell on it quietly. Why speak scriptures aloud? Because it's a powerful way to build our faith and often enables us to receive God's truth on a deeper level. Ask the Holy Spirit to shine new light on the verse for you. That's God's idea of meditation. Meditating on His Word and speaking it builds your faith, and you'll find yourself being transformed from the inside out! As Paul said, "We, who with unveiled faces all reflect the Lord's glory, are being transformed into His likeness" (2 Corinthians 3:18 NIV).

You can be transformed when you let the Word of God be your mirror instead of the physical looking glass on the wall or the poor reflection of the airbrushed wonder women on the covers of fashion magazines. Old thought patterns that don't line up with what God says about you are also false images of who you really are.

Do you want to release the gorgeous spiritual butterfly that's inside of you? Get away from the world and explore God's Word. Meditate on it and let the Holy Spirit change you on the inside. Then you'll begin to see changes on the outside, too. This is a prescription for perfection no pill, powder, or potion can match! Listening to Scripture read with soothing music in the background is also helpful.

A Heavenly Prescription

In Proverbs 4:20-22 we discover that God's words are "life to those who find them, and health to all their flesh." The Hebrew word for "health" (*marpê*) literally means "medicine." Speaking God's Word over your life is like taking daily doses of God's medicine—and you can never overdose on it! It's the method by which our faith grows. ("Faith comes by hearing, and hearing by the word of God").[11]

Since God's words are life and health, the more we meditate on them, the healthier and stronger we'll become spiritually, emotionally, and physically. We're agreeing with what God says about us instead of what the enemy says.

Did you know you can take control of your thoughts? You can! Whenever I catch myself worrying or dwelling on negative thoughts, Scripture reminds me to "[cast] down arguments and every high thing that exalts itself against the knowledge of God, bringing every thought into captivity to the obedience of Christ."[12] Like a big child, I will often reach up and act as if I'm grabbing a thought with my hand, throwing it to the ground, and stepping on it. "Gotcha!" I exclaim. "I refuse to entertain those thoughts."

Next step? I say one or several scriptures aloud that refute the negative thought. For example, after kicking out the whiny "I can't do it; this is too hard!" thought, I might quote Philippians 4:13: "I can do all things through Christ who strengthens me." Or I might speak a scriptural affirmation aloud. (A scriptural affirmation is a verse from the Bible spoken in the first person so you are applying it personally.)

As an experiment, I invite you to repeat the following scriptural affirmations right now and watch what happens. Speak them aloud, boldly declaring what your heavenly Father says about you: "I can do all things through Christ who strengthens me. I am strong in the Lord and in the power of His might. I am more than a conqueror through Him who loves me!"[13]

There! It's impossible to dwell on negative thoughts with those God-inspired, faith-filled words coming out of your mouth. Romans 12:2 tells us, "Do not conform any longer to the pattern of this world, but be *transformed by the renewing of your mind.*" That's exactly what you're doing when you declare the truth of God's Word to counter the lies and self-defeating thoughts Satan wants you to believe! The Holy Spirit will transform you from the inside out as you choose to pray in line with God's Word, think His thoughts (meditate on the Word), and boldly declare that no matter what your circumstances seem to say to the contrary, what God says is truth, and His truth will stand. As Paul stated,

> We do not look at the things which are seen, but at the things which are not seen. For the things which are seen are temporary, but the things which are not seen are eternal (2 Corinthians 4:18).

BUSY WOMAN'S QUICK TIPS
TRANSFORMERS FOR THE TONGUE

*Let the words of my mouth and the
meditation of my heart be acceptable in Your sight,
O LORD, my strength and my Redeemer.*
PSALM 19:14

Following are several scriptural affirmations (first-person declarations based on Scripture) that you can meditate on and speak aloud. Let their truths renew your mind and be transformed thereby!

I am strong in the Lord and in the power of His might (Ephesians 6:10).

The LORD is the strength of my life (Psalm 27:1).

My body is the temple of the Holy Spirit (1 Corinthians 6:19).

I present my body a living sacrifice, holy and acceptable to God, which is my reasonable service (Romans 12:1).

[Act this one out] I am taking up the whole armor of God that I may be able to stand in the evil day. I am girding my waist with truth. I've put on the breastplate of righteousness. I have shod my feet with the preparation of the gospel of peace. Above all, I am taking up the shield of faith so that I can quench all the fiery darts of the wicked one. I am putting on the helmet of salvation and taking up the sword of the Spirit, which is the word of God (Ephesians 6:13-17).

The Word of God is a lamp to my feet and a light to my path (Psalm 119:105).

He who is in me is greater than he who is in the world (1 John 4:4).

As I delight myself in the LORD, He will give me the desires of my heart (Psalm 37:4).

Some other important scriptural affirmations for Total Fitness are:

Wisdom is the principal thing; therefore I get wisdom. And In all my getting, I get understanding (Proverbs 4:7).

I give attention to God's words; I incline my ear to His sayings. I do not let them depart from my eyes; I keep them in the midst of my heart; for they are life to me, for I have found them, and they are health to all my flesh. I keep my heart with all diligence, for out of it spring the issues of life. I put away from me a deceitful mouth, and put perverse lips far from me (Proverbs 4:20-24).

I discipline my body and bring it into subjection, lest, when I have preached to others, I myself should become disqualified (1 Corinthians 9:27).

Yielding to the Fruit of the Spirit for Total Fitness

The heart of Total Fitness—spirit, soul, and body—is found in our relationship with God. Changing unwholesome habits, developing new ones, and experiencing joy on the journey all stem from our connection with Him. Lasting physical change doesn't result from diet or exercise alone but from allowing the Holy Spirit to develop His fruit in our lives ("love, joy, peace, patience, kindness, goodness, faithfulness, gentleness, and self-control")[14] as we yield to Him and walk in His power. As I mentioned earlier, I call this "yielding to the fruit of the Spirit." Our part is to allow the fruit of the Holy Spirit to be evident in our lives by choosing not to yield to our sinful nature and the works of the flesh.[15] Instead we yield to the fruit of the Spirit.

Yielding to the fruit of the Spirit takes mental decision and emotional willingness. For example, let's say you're standing in line at the grocery store, and an older gentleman is in front of you. The dear man is having a time of it—he can't find his glasses (on top of his head) so he can see to write a check (his checkbook fell on the floor), and he's misplaced the clerk's pen (it's in his pocket). You're late for an appointment and feel the pressure mounting inside as you tap your foot, glance at your watch, and clear your throat. Your flesh wants to scream, but the Holy Spirit sends you a gentle reminder about yielding to the fruit of patience in this situation. At one time you might have blurted out something unbecoming a lady, but you're different now. You decide, *Okay, I get it. This is an opportunity to let patience have its perfect work in me. I'm not going to get upset about this. Besides, it's by faith and patience that I inherit the promises of God, so all the good stuff I'm believing Him for is just that much closer to me now. Thank You, Lord.* Then you take out your cell phone and call the person your appointment is with to let her know you'll be a few minutes late. Lo and behold! She's running late too, and she is grateful you called.

A few years ago you would have let loose, but now you yield to patience as easily as you yield to love when your baby or grandchild makes a mess. You don't throw a wall-eyed fit when that happens, do you? Of course not. It's easy to yield to the fruit of love in that instance. If someone hurts your feelings, are you more likely to yield to love and forgive him or her now than you would have been several years ago?

Making changes in your life on the road to Total Fitness involves yielding to the fruit of the Spirit as well—primarily yielding to the fruit of patience, faithfulness, and self-control. *Patience* involves refusing to give up (one of the reasons it's also called "*long*suffering" in some versions!). *Faithfulness* is a steadfast determination to continue to show up for the appointments you make to spend time with the Lord, to exercise, to follow a sensible food plan, and to abide by any other fitness decisions you've made, such as being faithful to drink more water or eliminate certain foods or substances you know are harmful to you. *Self-control* in its simplest form is knowing when to say yes and when to say no, and acting on that knowledge.

The liberating truth about the fruit of the Spirit is that it's the fruit of the *Spirit* with a capital *S*. It's not *your* fruit! You don't have to drum it up or manufacture it out of the blue. The Lord offers us the fruit of the Spirit so we'll have strength to meet any situation. Our part is to choose to yield to Him, allowing Him to produce His fruit in our lives rather than going our own way. If you've discovered, as I have, that going your own way has caused "a world of hurt," as my country cousins would say, determine right now that you're ready to begin yielding to God's way of doing things. If you are, please write "Yes!" in the margin.

Busy women don't have time to wade through plans and programs that might or might not work. They also want lasting changes, not just quick fixes. So in the chapters that follow, we'll explore not only what science and health experts say are the best ways to achieve physical fitness but also what God's Word has to say.

In addition, we'll discover some time-saving nutrition and fitness tips, plus learn how to experience peace amid the stresses of our lives. We'll also uncover how to yield to spiritual virtues that will enable us to be strengthened in our walk with the Lord and experience benefits for spirit, soul, and body that can last a lifetime.

MAKING IT PERSONAL

(Answers to exercises for chapters 1–10 appear at the end of the book.)

1. I am a _____. I have a _____ and live in a _____.

2. After I committed my life to the Lord, I noticed changes in several areas of my life. (If you aren't a Christian but would like to know more, see the "Special Invitation" section at the end of this book.) There were a few sudden changes. I no longer...

   _____

   _____

   Instead, I wanted to _____

   _____

   There were also gradual changes over time, such as _____

   _____

   _____

   I realize that God is still working on me in these areas: _____

   _____

   _____

   I commit the following areas of my life to the Lord, asking Him to help me have victory in each one of them: _____

   _____

   _____

3. Romans 14:23 says, "Whatever is not from _____ is sin." I realize I haven't been walking by faith in these areas:

   _____

   _____

Lord, please forgive me. Help me walk by faith, trusting You.
I refuse to walk in doubt and unbelief.

4. Transformers for the tongue:

   Instead of saying (negative belief) _____

   _____,

   I will say (scriptural affirmation) _____

   _____.

   Instead of saying (negative belief) _____

   _____,

   I will say (scriptural affirmation) _____

   _____.

5. I believe the Lord is prompting me to focus on this aspect of the fruit of the Spirit more than any other right now: _____

   (In chapter 8, under "Sowing Seeds for an Abundant Harvest," we'll focus on ways we can nurture the fruit of the Spirit in our lives to help us make permanent lifestyle changes.)

QUICK NUTRITION TIPS

Why do you spend money for
what is not bread, and your
wages for what does not satisfy?
Listen carefully to Me, and eat what
is good, and let your soul delight
itself in abundance.

ISAIAH 55:2

As a busy woman, you may find yourself opting for fast-food or pre-packaged convenience foods that save time in the kitchen but may lack in nutrition. Are there healthier options available? Absolutely!

Why *do* we spend our money on so many things that really don't satisfy us—body, soul, or spirit? Looking at today's verse, Isaiah 55:2, from a physical perspective, a lot of the foods most people in Western cultures buy are highly processed "dead" foods. Some think differentiating between "dead" food and "live" food is ludicrous: "So, you want your turkey sandwich to gobble and run across the table, feathers and all?" Of course not!

What most nutritionists mean by "live" food is food that's as close to nature as possible, such as vegetables, fruits, whole grains, nuts, and seeds. These foods are harvested and the only processing they might go through is being cut, chopped, ground, or squeezed. You can usually tell what these live foods are by looking at them rather than having to read a label to figure out the ingredients. They come packaged in bright, beautiful, all-natural wrappers designed by God and don't contain any man-made chemicals, additives, or preservatives.

Dead food is highly processed with chemicals, hormones, artificial colors and flavors, preservatives, and other additives that prolong shelf life. (Shelf "life" is really a misnomer, isn't it?)

I like making the distinction this way: There's God-made food from nature's bounty, and there's man-made food from a giant factory. Yes, we can take man-made food back to its beginnings and find its God-made origins, but how many processes did it go through between its original state and your dinner table? Most dead food was once live food, but it has long since fallen prey to countless alterations to make it last as long as possible on store shelves.

Dead food also has the reputation of being highly addictive. Manufacturers add significant amounts of sugar (aka high-fructose corn syrup [HFCS], dextrose, glucose, maltose, and sucrose) to all kinds of products. Read the labels! One of the problems with these forms of sugars (especially high-fructose corn syrup) is that your brain doesn't recognize them as food, so your body doesn't get the signal to stop eating. It wants more and more and more! Your body also has to work harder to filter out and eliminate man-made substances from the dead foods you eat. The closer to God-made you eat, the easier foods are to digest.

For a more in-depth discussion of nutrition and choices for the busy woman, please see chapter 4: Quick and Safe Weight-Loss Tips.

An Inconvenient Convenience

But aren't processed foods more convenient? Yes and no. They're convenient for the moment, perhaps, but they're inconvenient over time when we consider the toll chemicals and preservatives can take on our bodies.

A healthy body that gets regular exercise and nutritious, God-made food is more likely to have a fully functioning immune system able to handle an occasional highly processed meal. Toxins are eliminated more readily instead of being stored in fat. And here's the interesting thing: The more God-made foods you eat, the more you crave processed foods.

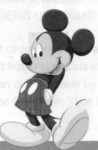

QUICK WOMAN'S QUICK TIP
THE DANGERS OF SUGAR

Following is an eye-opening list of some of the dangers of sugar. And this is only a partial list compiled from various medical and scientific sources. This list appeared in an online article by Dr. Nancy Appleton titled "Seventy-Six Ways Sugar Can Ruin Your Health."[1] Sugar has been shown to:

- suppress the immune system

- rapidly increase adrenaline levels, causing hyperactivity and moodiness in children

- increase triglycerides and bad cholesterol while lowering good cholesterol

- "feed" cancer cells

- weaken eyesight

- cause gastrointestinal problems

- cause dental problems, such as gum disease and tooth decay

- contribute to obesity, osteoporosis, and food allergies

- cause toxemia during pregnancy

- impair the structure of your DNA

- cause headaches, depression, and dizziness

- be addictive and intoxicating, like alcohol

Hopefully this information will lead you to consider choosing a replacement for this substance some consider as addictive as cocaine!

Today's busy woman doesn't have to sacrifice quality for convenience. Thankfully, there are options! Check out the following Nutritious Foods List and see how many live foods you can easily include in your diet (and your family's) on a regular basis. Are there some foods on the list you haven't tried before or haven't eaten in a long time? Are you willing to add a few to this week's menus?

THE NUTRITIOUS FOODS LIST

(preferably organic—no pesticides or preservatives)

Vegetables

Asparagus
Avocados
Beets
Bell peppers
Bok choy
Broccoli
Brussels sprouts
Cabbage (red and
    green)
Carrots
Cauliflower
Celery
Collard greens
Dandelion greens
Eggplant
Fennel
Garlic
Green beans
Green peas
Kale
Kelp and other sea
    vegetables
Leeks
Lettuce (leafy, not
    iceberg)
Mushrooms
Mustard greens
Olives
Onions
Parsley
Potatoes
Spinach
Squash (spaghetti,
    summer, winter)
Sweet potatoes
Swiss chard
Tomatoes
Turnip greens
Yams

Fruit

Apples
Apricots
Bananas
Blueberries
Cantaloupe
Cranberries
Dates
Figs
Grapefruit
Grapes
Kiwifruit
Lemons and limes
Mangoes
Oranges
Papaya
Peaches
Pears
Pineapple
Plums
Prunes
Raisins
Raspberries
Strawberries
Watermelon

Legumes
(Includes Beans)

Black beans
Chickpeas (garbanzo
    beans)

Kidney beans
Lentils
Lima beans
Miso (fermented soy)
Navy beans
Pinto beans
Soybeans
Tempeh (fermented soy)
Tofu (soy curd)

Nuts and Seeds

Almonds
Cashews
Flaxseed
Pecans
Pumpkin seeds
Sesame seeds
Sunflower seeds
Walnuts

Whole Grains

Barley
Brown rice
Buckwheat
Millet
Oats
Quinoa (pronounced "keen-wah")
Rye
Spelt (an ancient wheat)
Sprouted grain breads
Whole-grain pastas
Whole wheat

Fish and Seafood (Nonfarm Raised)

Cod
Halibut
Salmon (wild)
Snapper
Tuna

Poultry and Lean Meat

Beef (grass-fed, lean)
Buffalo
Chicken (hormone-free)
Turkey (hormone-free)

Dairy (Low-Fat and Hormone-Free)

Cheese (rice, soy, goat, cow)
Eggs (organic)
Milk (almond, rice, soy, goat, cow)
Yogurt (soy or dairy)

Good Fat (Includes Good Sources of Omega 3)

Almonds
Extra-virgin olive oil
Fish (such as salmon)
Flaxseed, pumpkin, or walnut oil (for dressings, and sauces)
Flaxseed, pumpkin

seeds, sunflower seeds
Omega 3 supplements
Walnuts and hazelnuts

Natural Sweeteners

Agave nectar
Blackstrap molasses
Honey
Maple syrup
Stevia
Xylitol

Other Healthful Products

Carob
Green powder (barley, kamut, spirulina, PraiseFast Super Greens—see Resources)
Green tea (decaffeinated)
Herbs and spices
Mustard (organic)
Olive oil (extra virgin)
Rooibos tea (South African)
Tamari soy sauce
Vegenaise, Nayonaise (product names)
Water (spring, purified)

When You Can, Buy Organic

The foods on the Nutritious Foods List were chosen because they provide the greatest amount of nutrients with the least amount of calories. The more of these foods you eat, the more disease-fighting, anti-aging phytonutrients (plant nutrients) and antioxidants your body will be receiving, in addition to vitamins, minerals, fibers, and essential fatty acids (EFAs). (EFAs play an important role in many metabolic processes and cardiovascular health. These "good fats" are essential and are different from trans fats, which are industrially created and have been linked to coronary disease.)

Whenever possible, choose organic foods. Yes, they cost more, but the upside is you'll receive the most nutrition possible without the chemical pesticides, synthetic fertilizers, antibiotics, or growth hormones found in conventional foods. We come across enough toxins in our day-to-day lives without ingesting them in our food supply! Quite frankly, as we understand the benefits of eating health-giving, live foods and the disadvantages of eating dead, chemical-laden foods, we'll be more willing to invest in our health up front instead of paying later when our health suffers. (If you're overcoming illness and rebuilding your health, take heart! Adding these nutritious foods to your diet will strengthen your body's natural disease-fighting abilities and can promote a quicker, more energetic recovery.)

Other benefits of organic food are that it's healthier for the soil and promotes the humane treatment of animals. You can consider yourself a better steward of God's creation by supporting companies that adhere to organic farming practices.

(When you have to buy nonorganic produce, make sure you wash them thoroughly. Spray with mixture of 1 T. lemon juice, 1 T. baking soda, and 1 C. water, and then rinse under running water.)

Planning Ahead

Making quality decisions ahead of time about meals will give you the upper hand against snack attacks and the perennial question, "What are we having for dinner?" Pick one evening a week to plan your menus and write your shopping list. Be sure to include fitness-friendly, ready-to-eat snacks. When you come home at the end of the day (and your husband and kids, if you're married), you'll be less tempted to make unwise snacking decisions if your kitchen is stocked with healthful snacks.

It's essential for your fitness success to have ready-made snacks available so you can reach for something quick when your blood sugar is low and your mind and will are a tad dull. Not many of us are willing to chop up some veggies when the "Three Musketeers" are calling our names!

Sensible Substitutes

One of the easiest ways to improve the nutritional value of the meals you and your family eat is to make health-conscious substitutions of low-fat, sugar-free, and organic foods for high-fat, sugary, and preservative-packed foods whenever possible. If the foods you tend to eat are highly processed (meaning they've gone through a number of processes from the time they left nature to when they reached your supermarket shelf), you're probably sacrificing nutrition and quality for convenience.

The good news is there are quick, inexpensive, and relatively painless upgrades you can make to your diet that will ensure you get the most nutrient-dense meals for the least amount of calories.

Do you have some favorite recipes you'd like to give a quick fitness makeover? Often low-fat, low-calorie ingredients can be substituted for high-fat or high-calorie ones. When cooking or baking, ask yourself how essential a particular ingredient is and see if a substitute will work. You'll wind up with a lower-calorie, heart-healthy version of an old favorite. You can also eliminate such nonessentials as salt and oil from the water when you cook pasta. Since they're not vital to the recipe, leave them out.

Reduce fat and sugar in your recipes by one-third to one-half by brushing a pan lightly with oil and wiping up the excess.

BUSY WOMAN'S QUICK TIP
THE SNACK ZONE

Make healthful foods convenient instead of opting for prepackaged "convenience" foods. Label a section on your kitchen counter, a shelf in your pantry, and a shelf in your refrigerator "The Snack Zone."

Keep a big bowl of fresh and dried fruits on the kitchen counter. Place a bowl of sliced, fresh fruit in the fridge. Go for seasonal favorites: Cut up fresh cantaloupe, honeydew melon, and strawberries one week; watermelon, grapes, and apples the next. Keep low-fat yogurt handy. Make good drinks easily accessible, such as homemade lemonade (with real lemons and good-for-you sweeteners like agave nectar, stevia, or xylitol), bottled water, or a big pitcher of herbal tea.

Here are more delicious and speedy snacks you and your family may enjoy:

- Low-fat yogurt as a dipping sauce or a topping on fruit salad.

- Cut up carrots, celery, red and green peppers, cauliflower, and broccoli.

- Low-fat sour cream, plain yogurt, or cheese dip for veggies and fruit.

- Whole-wheat flour tortillas filled with turkey or crumbled soy burger, low-fat dairy cheese or soy cheese, and lettuce. Wrap in foil and pop in the toaster oven to melt the cheese.

- Apple slices with 2 to 3 teaspoons of almond butter or no-sugar peanut butter spread on each slice.

- Apple slices with low-fat dairy cheese or soy cheese.

- Air-popped popcorn sprinkled with Mrs. Dash salt-free seasonings.

- Baked tortilla chips with salsa.

- Applesauce with raisins.

Here is a list of common ingredients and some sensible substitutes you can use.

1. *Sugar. Stevia* is a wonderful, good-for-you natural sugar substitute that can be used in baked goods and on cereals, as well as in hot or cold drinks. A member of the chrysanthemum family, it has zero calories, carbohydrates (carbs), and sugars. The sweet leaves from the stevia bush are available in liquid drops or powdered form at health-food stores and in some supermarkets.

Agave nectar is a slow-releasing carbohydrate sweetener that looks and tastes like honey yet has half the calories of sugar. While honey rates a 75 on the glycemic index (meaning it can really spike blood sugar), agave enters the bloodstream more slowly and registers at a low 11, making it more acceptable for diabetics and those of us interested in weight control.

Xylitol is the common name for a naturally occurring sugar called *xylose* that's derived from corncobs and birch bark. Although it has the sweetness of common sugar, it has 40 percent fewer calories and zero sugars. And since it's metabolized without insulin, it creates a lower glycemic effect, which is good news for diabetics. It's perhaps the only sweetener that can claim dental and antibacterial benefits and is endorsed by several European dental associations.

As with other dead foods, steer clear of man-made sugar substitutes.

2. *Eggs.* If a recipe calls for a whole egg, substitute two egg whites instead (preferably organic) or 1/4 cup of an egg substitute.

3. *Butter or margarine.* When browning vegetables, instead of adding butter, margarine, or oil to the pan first, put the vegetables in the pan, then spray them with oil. This reduces the amount of oil the vegetables can absorb during cooking.

If you're looking for a good butter or margarine replacement, try organic butter or nondairy, organic oil-blend spread, such as Earth

Balance whipped spread. (This is one that I can honestly say, "Wow! It tastes just like butter!")

4. *Oil.* Applesauce is a great substitute for oil, margarine, and butter in baked products, such as quick breads, muffins, and some cakes. Pureed prunes (like baby-food prunes) work as fat replacements in chocolate recipes, such as brownies and chocolate cake. Not only do the prunes retain moisture, but they also add richness to the color of baked goods. Substitute an equivalent amount of applesauce for the fat in the recipe.

5. *Fat (includes lard and shortening).* You can replace the fat in many recipes with an equal-volume mixture of half buttermilk and half applesauce. In recipes calling for beef, chicken, or vegetable stock, use vegetable or chicken bouillon cubes (preferably low-salt). When combined with water, bouillon cubes are a great low-calorie substitute. You can also add bouillon cubes and water to stir-fries to enhance flavor and reduce the amount of fat needed for cooking.

6. *Cheese.* Use 1/2 to 1 cup of lower-fat or reduced-fat cheese, such as part-skim mozzarella or ricotta, for every cup of cheese in a recipe. For casseroles, mix 1/2 cup of low-fat cottage cheese with 1/2 cup of reduced-fat cheese. For a nondairy substitute, try delicious soy-, rice-, or almond-milk cheeses, available in most health-food stores.

7. *Whole milk.* Using skim milk in place of whole milk reduces a recipe's fat content by 8 grams per cup! Nondairy options include soy, rice, or almond milk.

8. *Salad dressing.* There are many organic, low-calorie, low-fat, or nonfat options available now. Balsamic or organic apple-cider vinegar and olive oil or flaxseed oil are always healthful standbys. You

want to make sure you're getting good fats in your diet, and extra-virgin olive oil, ground flaxseed, and flaxseed oil definitely qualify. Fruit juice can be used to replace oil in low-fat salad dressings.

9. *Marinades.* Use fruit juice for a meat or vegetable marinade, or combine fruit juice with defatted chicken or vegetable broth for a less fruity marinade.

10. *Mayonnaise.* Low-fat or nonfat plain yogurt makes a good substitute, or mix 3/4 cup of plain yogurt with 1/4 cup or less of mayonnaise in your recipes. There are also good nondairy mayonnaise substitutes at your health-food store, such as Vegenaise and Nayonaise.

11. *Sour cream.* Again low-fat or nonfat yogurt comes to the rescue. You can make a good low-calorie version of sour cream by mixing 1 cup of low-fat cottage cheese, 2 tablespoons of buttermilk, and 1 teaspoon of lemon juice in a blender or food processor until smooth.

12. *Cream cheese.* Neufchâtel cheese or low-fat cream cheese or ricotta cheese work nicely.

13. *Cream.* In chowder recipes, puree half of the potatoes and other vegetables, then put them back into the chowder to create thickness and creaminess without having to use cream.

14. *Baking chocolate.* Use 3 tablespoons of cocoa powder for every ounce of baking chocolate. Carob (also called St. John's bread) is also a good replacement for chocolate, and it can be sweetened with stevia or xylitol.

15. *Bacon.* Turkey bacon or one of the textured vegetable-protein products (such as soy protein) are lower-fat substitutes for high-fat bacon.

16. *Ground beef.* Use extra-lean ground beef (10 percent fat or less) or select a lean cut of beef (preferably grass-fed) that you can ask your butcher to grind for you. Cuts such as round, sirloin, flank, and tenderloin are good choices. After cooking, drain all the fat and rinse the meat with hot water. When using ground beef in enchiladas or burritos, try reducing the amount of ground beef and adding mashed black or pinto beans instead. Soy substitutes are also very tasty and available in the frozen-foods section of most grocery stores. Some of these substitutes, such as Morningstar Farms Meal Starters Grillers Recipe Crumbles, have 80 percent less fat than ground beef.

17. *Pasta.* Most of us would admit if pressed that we love pasta. Yet few of us love pasta so much that we would eat it plain. That's because pasta is mainly used as a vehicle for flavorful sauces we enjoy. Regrettably, this particular vehicle is a starch that turns to sugar when we digest it. Since the flavor of the sauce is what we really want, let's use more nutritious vehicles with more flavor and fewer calories.

Try using different vegetables as replacements for starch. Spaghetti squash is great for replacing spaghetti. Strips of zucchini or yellow squash can be cut with a shredder or vegetable peeler to replace lasagna noodles.

If you absolutely must have pasta, try whole wheat, soybean, rice, spelt (an ancient wheat), or one of the other more healthful varieties. Average white pasta is bleached white flour and water. Remember making paste with flour and water in kindergarten? Pasta = paste. So use it with care.

18. *Potatoes.* Instead of having mashed potatoes, try pureed cauliflower. Another alternative is sweet potatoes. They're an excellent source of vitamins C and A and are loaded with antioxidants. They're also blood-sugar friendly, partly due to the fact they're about twice as high in dietary fiber than ordinary potatoes. Fiber slows digestion and the release of sugar into the bloodstream. The other reason has to do with their glycemic index, a ranking system for

carbohydrates based on their effect on blood-sugar levels during the first two or three hours after a meal. For example, the glycemic index for sweet potatoes is 54 versus a baked potato's rating of 93. The index values of a particular carbohydrate may vary depending on the variety (such as a baked Yukon-gold potato versus an Idaho baking potato) and how it's cooked. Carbohydrates that break down slowly, releasing glucose gradually into the bloodstream, have a low glycemic index. This is especially important for diabetics and anyone interested in weight loss.

19. *Corn chips and potato chips.* Crisped-rice and corn-flake cereals work well if you want to add a delectable crunch to casseroles or breadlike toppings. Reduced-fat or baked corn chips are another option.

Quick Round-the-Clock Tips

The following are some quick and easy meal suggestions for breakfast, lunch, and dinner, as well as a few tempting dessert and snack ideas:

Breakfast. Eggs are a great source of protein for breakfast and can be prepared any number of ways. I prefer egg whites to whole eggs, especially when I'm trying to lose extra pounds. Look for cage-free eggs or those with the USDA Organic label, which means that neither the hens nor their feed has been subjected to antibiotics, hormones, pesticides, or herbicides. Here are some fortifying breakfast ideas:

- Omelets are a quick-and-easy meal any time of day. Just add your favorite veggies, leftovers, meat, and vegetable-protein products. Try an egg-white omelet to reduce the amount of fat and cholesterol.

- Eggs can be scrambled, hard-boiled or soft-boiled, or poached. Add a side of whole-grain toast and a piece of fruit.

- How about a quick, low-fat quiche for dinner and left-overs for breakfast and lunch the next day?

- Cereal is always a favorite. Try whole-grain cereals, brown rice, oatmeal, and rye cereal—hot or cold—with almond milk or skim milk and your favorite fruit.

- Try whole-wheat or Ezekiel 4:9 brand of bagels, bread, or English muffins with all-fruit jam or almond butter. (Ezekiel 4:9 cites wheat, barley, lentils, millet, and spelt.)

- If you're eating a carbohydrate-rich breakfast (grains and breads, for example), you can slow the release of sugar into the bloodstream by adding a small amount of nuts or seeds (almonds, walnuts, macadamia nuts, sunflower seeds, etc.). The good fat found in nuts and seeds can help prevent blood-sugar imbalances by slowing the uptake of sugar into the bloodstream.

- Interested in a coffee substitute? Ask at your health-food store for Teeccino, a caffeine-free herbal coffee. Postum or Caffix are also pleasant-tasting, roasted-grain beverages.

Lunch. Focus on protein at lunchtime, along with a big veggie salad, to ensure stamina throughout the afternoon and avoid that midafternoon slump from overdoing carbohydrates. Combining different sources of protein in a salad (without loading up on fatty, chemical-laden salad dressing) is a smart choice for a high-powered lunch. Choose eggs, chicken, turkey, fish, or soy products. Here are a few ideas:

- Warmed whole-wheat tortillas stuffed with avocado, broccoli-slaw, shredded cheese (dairy, soy, or almond cheese), tomatoes, spinach leaves, and salsa is one of my favorite home lunches.

- Hard-boil one or two eggs and crumble them over a big leafy-green salad with veggies.

- Make a pot of homemade vegetable soup with bits of chicken or soy burger.

- Sandwiches are easy meals to prepare if you're on the go. Try chicken, egg, or tuna salad (light on the mayo) with spinach leaves, romaine, or green leaf lettuce on whole-grain or Ezekiel 4:9 bread or rolls.

- If you decide to eat out, eat as many whole, unprocessed foods as possible for maximum fitness and energy. Salad bars are a great choice. Stick to small portion sizes instead of all-you-can-possibly-eat-until-you-fall-over heapin' helpings. Load up on the greens, but go light on the dressing.

- If you're craving Mexican food, enjoy tortillas, enchiladas, fajitas, and quesadillas with beans or meat (but light on the cheese). Avoid white rice and fried tortilla chips.

- *Brown-bag tips:* Prepare lunches the night before to avoid the last-minute morning rush. If you have children, limit portion sizes to avoid waste (1/2 cup servings, half a sandwich, a few fruit slices instead of the whole fruit, and baby carrots). Provide a vegetable and a protein with each meal (proteins include lean meats, soy products, whole grains and beans combined, nut butters, or nuts and seeds combined). (Nuts and seeds together or beans and whole grains combined constitute what's called a "complete protein.") Include a sugar-free treat in each lunch (fruit, applesauce-snack container, raisins, homemade cookies, a muffin). Keep moist sandwich ingredients in a separate container to avoid soggy sandwiches.

Dinner. Remember the adage "Eat the breakfast of a king, the lunch of a prince, and the dinner of a pauper"? Dinner should be your smallest meal of the day. Eat more protein and less carbohydrates to lose weight. Try any of the following meal suggestions:

- Many of the lunch suggestions will also work for dinner. Even some breakfast items make a nourishing dinner, such as an omelet or a quiche with a side salad of veggies and brown rice.

- Stir-fry veggies with a little olive oil and a protein source (such as soy crumbles, chicken, or fish). Serve with whole-wheat pasta or brown rice and salad. Don't forget to add those fresh sprouts!

- Mix up a pot of chili (with or without meat) and serve with brown or basmati rice and lightly steamed or raw veggies.

- If you want to have pasta for dinner, try chicken with a tomato-based sauce on whole-wheat pasta with salad.

- Instead of hamburgers, make turkey burgers, serve with baked sweet potato and shredded cabbage-carrot slaw.

- Avoid table salt. Use sea salt or seasonings without mono-sodium glutamate (MSG), such as Mrs. Dash. You might also experiment with fresh herbs from the supermarket—or grow your own!

Desserts and snacks. Retrain your taste buds to enjoy the natural sweetness of fresh fruit without sugar or artificial sweeteners. Enjoy these tasty treats anytime:

- Garnish a fresh fruit salad with a sprig of mint.

- Instead of chocolate, ask for carob powder or carob chips at your health-food store. (It's sometimes called St. John's bread.) Carob is similar to chocolate but without the sugar or caffeine.

- Peel a banana, cut it into slices, and freeze the slices in wax paper or a freezer bag. I enjoy this treat with carob chips. A variation is to dip a banana in melted carob chips, place it on wax paper, and freeze it. You can also poke a popsicle stick into one end of the banana (before freezing) for a delectable banana-carob pop.

- Wash and freeze grapes for an icy treat on a hot day.

- Whip up a fruit smoothie for a filling and healthful snack.

Good Fast Food?

Is there such a thing as *good* fast food? Well, let's hope so, since we can't always eat at home or take food with us, especially when we're traveling. Americans spend more than $110 billion on fast food every year (up from $6 billion in 1970). That's more money than we spend on personal computers, higher education, or new cars! Many health experts blame fast food and lack of exercise for the startling rise in obesity in America. Studies indicate that 1 in 3 adults are overweight, and childhood obesity has tripled over the past 25 years.

Thankfully, menus are changing for the better at many fast-food restaurants. Fueled by consumer concerns, some of the popular burger chains have announced a policy of moving toward beef produced without hormones and antibiotics. Salads and meatless entrées are options in more places, and fruit salad with low-fat yogurt now offers a delightful alternative to the sugary, nondairy, frozen "What was that anyway?" treat in some restaurants.

Here are some smart choices to look for at your local drive-through café:

- Choose fresh salad, roasted or baked meats, nonfried foods.

- Steer clear of heavy sauces, cheese, mayonnaise, and bacon, which pack on the calories, fat, and cholesterol.

- Avoid creamy dressings, croutons, and fried tortilla shells with that salad.

- Opt for fat-free dressing on the side. (You can dip your fork into the dressing before skewering a leafy green, which gives you all the taste with minimal calories.)

- Say no to fried foods. Choose grilled, broiled, baked, or steamed entrées instead.

- Order chicken, turkey, or fish, which are leaner than ground beef.

- If you don't want to look supersized, don't order supersized! Choose a regular or junior meal with a salad on the side.

- Opt for roast-turkey, chicken, or veggie wraps (no cheese or mayo).

- Burritos without cheese or sour cream are also a relatively healthful choice.

- Try whole-wheat pita pockets stuffed with veggies or order Greek kebobs.

- Is there a Japanese restaurant nearby? Ask for a *bento box* (a more elegant equivalent to the American brown bag) with lean meat, veggies, rice, and fruit slices. Be sure to ask for low-sodium soy sauce.

- Chili, scrambled eggs, and vegetable soup are options in many places now too.

- Water is always the healthier choice over a 32-ounce soda.

- For breakfast on-the-go, choose scrambled eggs or an egg-and-English-muffin-style breakfast sandwich with a piece of fruit. Give the high-fat bombs a wide berth (like croissants, biscuits and gravy, bacon, and sausage biscuits).

- A baked potato with salsa and salad is a nutritious, filling choice.

- Is everyone going out for pizza? First, fill your plate with healthful choices at the salad bar. (Remember to have the low-fat dressing on the side.) Drink water with lemon. Then when the pizza comes, you'll be less likely to eat too much. One slice of pizza with low-fat cheese, tomato sauce, and a vegetable topping is a relatively good choice.

BUSY WOMAN'S QUICK TIP
YOU CAN TAKE IT WITH YOU!

Restaurant portions are larger than anyone can comfortably eat, especially those who are striving to maintain a healthy weight, let alone lose weight. Play it smart and decide that you won't allow temptation to get the best of you. When ordering at a restaurant, ask your server to put half of the entrée in a take-home carton *before* the meal is brought to you. Then eat the smaller amount on your plate. You probably won't be tempted to open the container and eat the other half. This will not only supply a meal for the next day but will be a blessing to your waistline and conscience as well.

The Most Important Meal of the Day

Are you a breakfast eater? It's important to eat a nutritious breakfast every morning if you want to maintain a good energy level throughout the day and either lose weight or maintain a healthy weight. One thing many overweight people have in common is they seldom eat breakfast. Consequently they start the day at a loss—a loss of energy, brain power, and memory, as well as a 5 percent drop in metabolism. People who don't eat breakfast also have a built-in trigger designed to cause overeating later in the day.

In 1992 Vanderbilt University conducted a study of overweight people who routinely skipped breakfast. When they began eating breakfast, they became big *losers,* losing an average of 17 pounds in 12 weeks. They were less hungry at other meals, and eating breakfast fired up their metabolisms to burn more fat the rest of the day.[2]

Breakfast = break fast. We're to break (or end) the fast (abstinence from food) we've been on since the last meal (or snack) we ate the night before. I like to see this as a command: Break your fast! Nutritionists and dietitians recommend eating your first meal of the day *no later* than one hour after awakening. If you're not hungry in the morning, the reason may be eating late the night before and going to bed with undigested food in your stomach. I often woke up groggy and "hungover" after a late-night food binge. The next morning the last thing I wanted to look at was food. Only around ten o'clock would something like a doughnut or sugary muffin sound appealing. But delaying or skipping breakfast can start a vicious cycle. If you hate eating breakfast like I did, it's possible that your blood chemistry is out of balance first thing in the morning. Breakfast may be just what your body needs to stabilize your blood sugar and stop a queasy stomach.

Digestive Problems?

If you have digestive problems (indigestion, gas, bloating, irritable-bowel syndrome, constipation, etc.), don't eat fruit with other foods. Try eating fruit first, wait 20 minutes, and eat the rest of your meal. Fruit digests quickly and will also help with elimination. Also avoid eating starches (such as bread or potatoes) with protein (such as eggs or meat). (You can eat them at separate meals.) Although God created us with the ability to digest many types of foods, if you're suffering from digestive problems, the combinations of foods you're eating may be the culprit. If your body isn't digesting food properly, you're probably not absorbing the nutrients from your food and your dietary supplements as you should, which can affect your general health and energy.

If you suspect food allergies or sensitivities, try eliminating wheat, coffee, tea, dairy, soy, corn, sugar or artificial sweeteners, and MSG from your diet for a month. Seek out a good nutritionist or dietitian who can help you design a nutritious diet you can enjoy. Also try the following Cleansing Breakfast for a few days and see if that helps you overcome some or all of your digestive problems.

BUSY WOMAN'S QUICK TIP
EASY, QUICK-ENERGY BREAKFASTS

How can you put together a delicious and nutritious breakfast if you're on a tight schedule or a tight budget—or both? It's as easy as 1, 2, 3 for quick energy!

1. Simple carbohydrate (such as juice, fresh or dried fruit) = Fast-start energy

2. Complex carbohydrate (such as whole-grain cereal or bread, but no white-flour products) = Sustained energy

3. Protein (such as eggs, meat, low-fat dairy, nuts, seeds, or soy) = Muscle-building energy

Here are a few examples:

(1) 1/2 banana + (2) 2/3-cup whole-grain cereal + (3) 1/2-cup skim milk

(1) orange juice + (2) 1 slice whole-grain toast + (3) 2 scrambled eggs

(1) all-fruit jam + (2) 1 whole-wheat muffin + (3) 1 tablespoon almond or peanut butter

Get the idea? Now you try it. Think of what you have available in the kitchen right now and write down two easy combinations you can have for breakfast tomorrow morning that you (and the rest of the family) will enjoy. Remember, "It's as easy as 1, 2, 3 for quick energy!"

(1) _____ + (2) _____ + (3) _____

(1) _____ + (2) _____ + (3) _____

If your meal doesn't have fat, add a small pat of butter, a few almonds, or consider your EFA supplement as fat for the meal.

Cleansing Breakfast

Whether or not you're experiencing digestive problems, another option for breakfast is to eat fruit and to drink freshly extracted vegetable juice for the first part of the day. Many health experts believe this helps the body go through a cleansing cycle. A good juicer is worth the investment, and your body will benefit from the concentrated nutrition.

Within an hour of rising in the morning, enjoy a cup of fresh, organic carrot juice or carrot-apple juice. (Your health-food store should be able to get you large, organic, juicing carrots.) Add a scoop of concentrated powdered greens for extra nourishment, such as PraiseFast Super Greens (see Resources).

Around nine o'clock (or shortly before leaving for the day if you work outside the home) take several fiber-supplement capsules or drink 2 to 3 tablespoons of freshly ground flaxseed or psyllium-seed husks added to juice or water to aid bowel function.

Around ten o'clock have a piece of fresh fruit (such as grapefruit, a peach, an apple, or an orange) to keep your energy up while your body is cleansing itself of harmful substances. Eating a light meal of fruit often helps people feel light and focused and is a healthful alternative to a heavy, fat-laden breakfast, such as biscuits and gravy, or a speedy, poor-quality choice, such as doughnuts and coffee. You'll also be aiding your digestive system as it cleanses itself during the first part of the day and giving your cells the nutrition they need.

Many women prefer staying on the Cleansing Breakfast plan for a prolonged period, while others follow it just a few days a week. Try it and see how you feel.

MAKING IT PERSONAL

1. Three foods from the Nutritious Foods List that I haven't eaten before or in a long time are _____, _____, and _____. I want to try them this week.

2. Following are unhealthy snacks I've been eating. I'd like to eat them less often and substitute more healthful foods for them.

   I will substitute _____ for _____.

   I will substitute _____ for _____.

   I will substitute _____ for _____.

3. I'm going to try some different healthful meals for breakfast, lunch, and dinner. One day this week I'll try _____ _____ for breakfast, on another day I'll try _____ for lunch, and one day I'll try _____ for dinner.

4. At my favorite fast-food restaurant, instead of _____, I'll try this more healthful choice: _____.

THE BEST MIRACLE
ELIXIR FOR THE MONEY

The earth was without form, and void;
and darkness was on the face of the deep.
And the Spirit of God was hovering
over the face of the waters.

GENESIS 1:2

There are so many choices available when it comes to beverages. Unfortunately not all of them are good for you. In fact, a dangerous trend is emerging in the United States: People are drinking soft drinks for breakfast!

The busy woman often finds herself eating and drinking on the go. According to data compiled by the NDP Group, a consumer market-research firm, soft-drink consumption with breakfasts eaten away from home "has nearly doubled in the past 15 years," while drinking coffee with breakfasts eaten away from home "has fallen nearly 25 percent."[1] These figures reflect only soft drinks consumed with meals and don't include coffee consumption at coffee-a-ramas, such as Starbucks, Caribou Coffee, and Java Dave's.

Most morning pop drinkers prefer regular soda, but diet-soda consumption is growing. According to the NPD Group, "Diet soda accompanied 1.7 percent of breakfasts in 1990." By 2006, "5.3 percent of those eating breakfast away from home had a diet pop, while 9.8 percent had a regular soda."[2] *U.S. News and World Report* stated that "since 1950, soft-drink consumption per capita has quadrupled, from about 11 gallons per year to about 46 gallons in 2003—nearly a gallon a week per person."[3]

It's all about getting that jolt of caffeine into the body the quickest way possible. And with the adrenal-pumping caffeine come other questionable additives. One can of regular soda has about 10 teaspoons of sugar, 150 calories, and 30 to 55 milligrams of caffeine, as well as artificial food colors and sulphites. "But," you say, "I drink *diet* soda." This may sound like a healthier alternative to regular pop, but some nutritional experts believe that artificial sweeteners in diet soda are worse than sugar, and they may actually make you crave more sweets and fattening foods.

The findings of recent studies published in the *International Journal of Obesity* showed that eating and drinking artificially sweetened foods and beverages may be causing people to underestimate their caloric intake. Laboratory animals consumed *three times more calories* than those that did not ingest artificial sweeteners.[4] Obesity rates in children seem to be linked to sodas as well. A study published in the *Lancet,* Britain's prestigious medical journal, states that for every soft drink or sugar-sweetened beverage a child drinks each day, his or her obesity risk jumps 60 percent.[5]

Not only are regular and diet sodas linked to the growing obesity epidemic, but soft-drink consumption has been linked to liver damage,[6] diabetes,[7] and mental-health problems,[8] while also exposing your body to toxic levels of benzene. (The Food and Drug Administration [FDA] has acknowledged that benzene, a carcinogen, has been found in U.S. soft drinks at levels above the limit considered safe for tap water.)[9]

Healthful Alternatives to Soda Pop

Ready to leave carbonated beverages behind but looking for a good substitute or an interim drink on your way to "Water, please, with a slice of lemon"? One way to enjoy the "fizzy" of carbonation without the sugar is to buy a two-liter bottle of soda water (carbonated without sugar) and half-gallon bottles or cans of 100 percent fruit-juice drinks (no added sugar). Mix the soda water and juice half and half in two liter bottles. Try different combinations for unique treats.

From there, move on to sparkling water with natural flavors (no sugar or artificial sweeteners). You can always sweeten sparkling water with flavored liquid stevia. Sparkling water with toffee-flavored stevia drops tastes like root beer. Lemon-flavored stevia with sparkling water makes a delightful lemony soda without the calories, sugars, carbohydrates, or chemicals of other sweeteners.

The day may come when you'll prefer purified water to any other beverage, but you can always enjoy a refreshing, healthful beverage for a change.

Coffee substitutes? As I mentioned in chapter 2, Teeccino is a delicious coffee alternative made from herbs, grains, fruits, and nuts that are roasted, ground, and brewed like coffee. The potassium in Teeccino gives your body a natural energy lift without the caffeine. Caffeine-free green tea is also delicious, as are other herbal teas served hot or cold with stevia, honey, xylitol, or agave nectar.

Water: The Miracle Elixir

Water is the number one God-made thirst quencher. More than half of your body is made up of water, and each part of the body contains different amounts. For example,

- Your muscles are about 75 percent water.
- Your brain is about 75 percent water.
- Your blood is about 82 percent water.
- Your bones are approximately 25 percent water. (No "dry bones," please!)

Water is a vital part of *every* bodily function, including breathing, eating, movement, circulation, temperature regulation, and brain activity. Amazingly, every 24 hours your remarkable God-made body recycles the equivalent of *40 thousand glasses* of water. And this is just to maintain normal physiological functions. A deficit of 6 to 10 glasses of water has to be replaced or dehydration (depletion of body fluids) will occur.

The good news is that you get about 1 quart (32 ounces) of water from the foods you eat *if* you eat plenty of fruits and vegetables. However, if your main food sources are starchy processed foods, cooked meats, and fats, you'll need to consume *more* water because these foods contain very little.

If you drink coffee, tea, or soft drinks, you need to drink *more* water because these caffeinated substances dehydrate the body, removing more water than the beverages actually contain. A good rule of thumb is to drink one 8-ounce glass above your normal water intake for every caffeinated drink you have. Of course, a better option would be to let go of the caffeine. Okay, I can tell I hit a nerve! Seriously though, you may find you feel better without the caffeine. Yes, you may experience withdrawal symptoms the first day or two when you don't get your "fix." (That alone is a good clue caffeine is addictive!) But once your body adjusts, it will thank you.

I know when I first gave up caffeine (and I did so on more than one occasion), I experienced a headache for the first day, but then I felt a lot more clear-headed after that.

BUSY WOMAN'S QUICK TIP
HOW MUCH WATER IS RIGHT FOR YOU?

Most people don't drink enough water every day to stay properly hydrated. In general, it's important to drink at least eight to ten 8-ounce glasses of water each day. A better way to determine how much water you need is by dividing your body weight in half. This gives you the amount of water you need in ounces every day. For example, someone who weighs 150 pounds needs 75 ounces of water daily. (That's just over nine 8-ounce glasses of water). An easy way to keep track of your water intake would be to fill a 36-ounce travel mug with purified water and drink a little more than two full mugs each day.

BUSY WOMAN'S QUICK TIP
COFFEE—WHAT'S THE GOOD NEWS ON THE OLD GRIND?

Is there anything good about coffee? Yes! Since caffeine boosts metabolism, it is often a primary ingredient in weight-loss formulas. Recent studies, including those at both Harvard and Vanderbilt University's Institute for Coffee Studies, have found that coffee may help prevent Parkinson's disease and cirrhosis of the liver. It may also lower risks for developing type-two diabetes, colon cancer, high blood pressure in women, and heart disease. Part of the reason may be that coffee is loaded with more than 1,000 antioxidants (more than green tea!).

Call me a skeptic, but I think it's more than a little interesting that the Institute for Coffee Studies has received funding from Kraft Foods (makers of Maxwell House coffee), the Association of Coffee Producing Countries (Brazil and Colombia), a coalition of Central American coffee-producing nations, the National Coffee Association of the USA, and the All Japan Coffee Association.[10] No conflict of interest there, eh?

If you're a busy woman experiencing any of the following symptoms, I strongly urge you to consider kicking the caffeine habit:

- difficulty sleeping
- restlessness
- jitteriness
- anxiety
- nausea
- flushed face
- fibrocystic breasts
- uterine fibroids
- headaches
- accelerated heartbeat or heart arrhythmias

Many women who suffer from painful periods caused by uterine fibroids (fibroid tumors), which are benign 99 percent of the time, notice a marked improvement in their monthly cycles when they eliminate caffeine from their diets.

Don't Wait Until You're Thirsty!

Dehydration is an all-too-common condition, but most of us aren't even aware of this very real danger. By the time you feel thirsty, your body may already be dehydrated. And once you're dehydrated, your endurance is diminished, strength can drop, and the negative effects can last for a day or more (something a busy woman does *not* need!). Other symptoms of dehydration can include dizziness, headache, irritability, dry mouth, cramps, and flushed skin.

Your body loses a lot of water each day:

- Sixteen ounces through respiration (on average)

- Sixteen ounces through invisible perspiration, such as through the feet (more if perspiration is visible)

- Forty-eight ounces through elimination (The more food you eat, the more water will be lost with additional elimination.)

Instead of relying on a thirst signal, drink water at regular intervals whether you're thirsty or not. Drink water cold when possible. Cold water absorbs into your body more quickly than warm water. Some experts also believe drinking cold water helps burn more calories.

I put a gallon of purified water in the refrigerator at night before I go to bed, knowing I plan to drink all or most of it the next day. Although it's double the half-your-body-weight-in-ounces formula for me, water is the only beverage I drink consistently.

Be sure to drink more water when exercising to avoid dehydration. (Keep a bottle of it with you at the gym or have one within easy reach immediately before and after a brisk walk.) Drink more water in warm weather or when you're working outdoors. I keep bottled water in my car so I can keep drinking while I'm driving around town.

Where Dehydration Can Lead

The Lord designed the human body in such a way that if it detects dehydration, it will make sure that five vital organs always have adequate supplies of water to function, even if it means taking water from the other systems. These five vital organs are the heart, lungs, kidneys, brain, and liver. Water is needed to carry nutrients to these organs. Remember that your brain is about 75 percent water, and the blood that pumps through your heart is approximately 82 percent water. A shortage of water can cause a loss of water volume in the cells of these organs. This affects the body's ability to deliver nutrients to the cells and remove waste products, resulting in a deficiency of nutrients and a buildup of waste in the cells.

Chronic dehydration can lead to a host of debilitating conditions, including neck and back pain, arthritis and other kinds of joint pain, kidney stones, and high blood pressure. Does that seem hard to believe? Well, consider neck or back pain. Pain can be caused by discs wearing out because of insufficient fluid within the disc. Cartilage, the material between bones, is about 80 percent water. It provides a smooth surface that allows the joints to glide easily during movement. It's very slick—about five times slicker than ice. Well-hydrated cartilage ensures minimal frictional forces and allows the joints to remain healthy. Dehydrated cartilage increases frictional forces, which results in more damage to the cartilage and can lead to joint pain and possibly arthritis. Arthritis literally means an inflammation (*itis*) of the joints (*arthr*).

What do we often do when we experience pain? Drink water? Well, if we do, it's only enough to swallow a couple of aspirin or another painkiller.

Try looking at it this way: Arthritis and back pain aren't the result of a lack of aspirin or ibuprofen. So why do we take those products for pain? We take them to cover it, of course. But what if the solution was as simple as increasing our pure-water intake?

Now what about knee and other joint pain? Like the discs and cartilage in your neck and back, your joints need fluid to ensure proper movement. Synovial fluid, which is mostly water, lubricates and cushions your joints during movement. (The word "synovial" comes from the Latin word for "egg," referring to the egglike consistency of this fluid.) Synovial fluid is also important for joint function because it reduces the friction between the cartilage. If you become dehydrated, less synovial fluid is available to protect your joints and damage can occur.

I recently was experiencing pain in my knees while doing research for this book. Although I wasn't doing anything different, I realized I had slacked off on my daily water consumption. I've since increased my water intake and have noticed a marked improvement in both my knees.

What does dehydration have to do with high blood pressure or kidney stones? As mentioned, the body rations water to ensure that the vital organs (the brain, heart, kidneys, liver, and lungs) receive sufficient amounts. Hypertension (high blood pressure) is often caused by chronic dehydration. When you become dehydrated, your arteries may constrict (become narrow), limiting the flow of blood and water to other parts of the body so that your heart can pump blood to the vital organs first. When arteries become constricted, your blood pressure increases (similar to increasing water pressure by constricting a hose). Dehydration can also lead to thicker blood.

If you're concerned about high blood pressure, see your health-care provider or a qualified health professional who will work with you in the areas of nutrition and lifestyle changes. You may also want to significantly reduce the amount of salt or sodium you use in your food or switch to a salt substitute (like Mrs. Dash), since high sodium intake can cause high blood pressure. Some health experts advise avoiding all foods containing simple sodium or sodium chloride (processed salt). Sodium chloride isn't real salt. Instead, look for Celtic salt or sea salt. This is actual salt from the ocean, which is quite complex in its molecular structure and has a far different effect on your body than sodium chloride.

Dehydration is also one of the leading causes of excruciatingly painful kidney stones. Kidney stones are combinations of protein and various minerals (such as calcium, magnesium, or phosphate) that occur within the kidney or anywhere along the urinary tract. Interestingly, kidney stones are more common problems in the summer than during any other season. Health professionals believe this is because people are more active during the summer, perspiring more and becoming dehydrated more quickly. Although kidney stones affect 1 in 10 Americans, the simplest way to avoid them is to stay hydrated.

As I mentioned earlier, the general guideline for daily water consumption is eight to ten 8-ounce glasses of water. Studies indicate that drinking just five glasses of water daily decreases the risk of colon cancer by 45 percent, the risk of breast cancer by 79 percent, and the risk of developing bladder cancer by 50 percent.

Are you drinking the amount of water you need every day?

Looking to Lose Fat? Drink More Water!

Drinking a sufficient amount of water daily plays an important role in weight loss and healthy weight maintenance too. Decreasing water intake causes fat deposits to increase, and *increasing* water intake can reduce them. Why? The kidneys need water to function properly. When they aren't receiving sufficient water, they're not operating at full capacity, which means that some of the load has to be managed by the liver. One of the liver's many functions is to convert stored fat into energy, but if it's doing some of the work the kidneys are supposed to do, it's not able to function at maximum capacity. The result? The body stores more fat instead of metabolizing it.

Many women have told me they are rarely thirsty. This may be due to a physical imbalance. We can actually lose our natural thirst for water when our bodies become imbalanced from eating food when we're really thirsty or from drinking caffeinated soda, coffee, or tea, which further dehydrates the body.

You can regain your natural thirst by giving your body the water it craves (yes, even if you think you aren't thirsty). If you drink one quart of water over a 30-minute period in the morning, then another quart at noon, and again in the early evening, you'll hydrate your body, diminish water retention, and free your liver to metabolize stored fat. Your natural thirst will come back—perhaps for the first time in years. You may even discover that water has become your beverage of choice. After all, it is the God-made drink!

BUSY WOMAN'S QUICK TIP
HUNGRY? DRINK WATER

Would you believe that sometimes you only *think* you're hungry? You may actually be thirsty. I call it "mouth hunger." I experienced that sensation whenever I wanted something to eat, but the desire wasn't coming from my stomach. It would often be a taste in my mouth I wanted to change, and I knew that eating a certain snack would accomplish that. When I began drinking water instead of soda, juice, coffee, or tea, I found I wasn't hungry anymore. (I hadn't really been hungry to begin with. My body was crying out for water.) People who "graze" or snack all day will often lose weight if they drink water instead of eating when they experience mouth hunger.

Water Can Relieve Edema

Many women think that drinking the daily recommended amount of water will lead to bloating and swollen ankles. Actually, the opposite is typically the case. When the body isn't receiving enough water, it determines that dehydration is a threat to survival and retains water as a precaution, storing it in spaces outside the cells. This results in swollen ankles, feet, and hands. Drinking sufficient quantities of water often relieves this edema.

Diuretics only make things worse. Stored water may be forced out of the body for a time (along with minerals and other essential nutrients), but the body will replace the lost water as soon as it can. When the swelling returns and you take diuretics again, the cycle will repeat itself. If water retention is a problem for you, first try increasing your water intake and decreasing the amount of salt and caffeine in your diet rather than using a diuretic.

Water Filtration Options

Please don't drink tap water if at all possible. The water you use to wash your clothes, water the lawn, and flush the toilet shouldn't be used as drinking water. In a *New York Times* article it was reported that "more than 1 in 5 Americans unknowingly drink tap water polluted with feces, lead, radiation, or other contaminants."[11] Many large bottled-water companies simply filter tap water, so the exotic names and price tags mean little. You might as well filter your own! If you do purchase bottled water, spring water is a good choice. Mountain Valley Spring Water retains a natural mineral content consisting mainly of calcium, potassium, and magnesium. Its alkaline content is closer to the body's natural pH, so it helps you maintain a more alkaline balance. Drinking alkaline water also helps you keep enough healthy oxygen available to your blood cells. Penta water, available in health-food stores, undergoes a 13-step purification process and is considered by many to be the purest water on the market.

At home my family uses a Waterwise water purifier, which combines a steam distillation process with carbon filtration. It's believed that distilled water may make the body more acidic, so we usually add a couple teaspoons of organic apple-cider vinegar to a glass of distilled water to help regulate the body's pH balance.

Reverse-osmosis filters, alkaline filters, or inexpensive carbon filters are also good choices and are infinitely more beneficial to the body than tap water.

"I Hate Water!"

I'm amazed at how many women tell me they hate water. Others sheepishly admit they don't drink all the water they should. I can relate to the first group. I used to hate water, but then I read all the good things water does for the human body. I also realized that water is a symbol (or "type") of the Holy Spirit, mentioned 396 times in the Bible. Jesus said He'd give believers the *water* of life, not the Diet Coke, iced tea, or even orange juice of life.

Don't like the taste of water? Filtration systems can do wonders, and refrigerating water also helps improve the taste. You might try adding a squeeze of lemon or two teaspoons of organic apple-cider vinegar and a teaspoon of honey.

MAKING IT PERSONAL

1. _____ of my body is made up of water.

2. How much water should I drink each day? A good rule of thumb is half my _____ _____ in ounces. Starting today I will start drink at least _____ ounces of water each day.

3. Chronic dehydration can lead to a host of debilitating conditions, including _____, _____, _____, and _____.

4. On a daily basis, I drink about _____ cups of coffee, _____ cups/glasses of hot tea or iced tea, _____ cans/bottles of soft drinks, _____ glasses of juice, _____ glasses of milk, and _____ glasses of water.

5. I purpose to drink less _____ and more water.

6. One way I can be sure I drink the recommended amount of water each day is to _____ _____.

QUICK AND SAFE WEIGHT-LOSS TIPS

I call heaven and earth as witnesses
today against you, that I have set before
you life and death, blessing and curs-
ing; therefore choose life, that both you
and your descendants may live.

DEUTERONOMY 30:19

Choose Life to Experience Positive Change

Choose life! This is by far one of the quickest ways to experience positive change in our lives. Does it work for weight management, fitness, and vibrant health as well? Yes! The "choose life" decision can be made in a minute and lived out moment by moment one day at a time.

Why start a chapter about weight loss with a scriptural directive to choose life? As busy women, we need some practical, proactive tools we can use at a moment's notice to help us handle the decisions, challenges, and temptations we face in our Total Fitness journey. I've found that these simple yet startlingly powerful words keep me from falling prey to sudden urges for "just one" (as in just one bite, cookie, candy bar, missed walk, or exercise session).

You may be different, but for me "just one" rarely ends with just one. However, when I stop and say to myself, "Choose life," my spirit rises up with strength to overcome my flesh, and I'm able to say no to the temptation. I've also used these two potent little words from Scripture to get me moving when my flesh wants to "veg out" in front of the television or skip the walk I've committed to take. "I choose life," I'll say as I lace up my running shoes and head for the door or the mini-trampoline. "I choose life" I've said to myself when I've wanted to pout and punish my husband for hurting my feelings instead of forgiving him. Choosing to follow those three little words often turns the whole situation around.

Do I use these words as some sort of magic incantation or lucky charm? No, certainly not. Magic and luck are part of the enemy's bag of tricks. When you have the blessing and favor of God through your relationship with Jesus Christ, you want nothing to do with capricious fortune, magic, or luck. God's promises are based on truth, not happenstance.

What "Choose Life" Means

We're presented with hundreds, even thousands, of choices every day that affect the health and fitness of our spirits, souls, and bodies. How well I know the cry of the flesh, "I want it, and I want it *now!*" I always had to have my favorite snack or drink or a second helping—my "fix." Like a child I thought only of the desire of the present moment and wanted to have my own way. Let the grown-ups deal with the consequences. It didn't matter how strong my willpower had been moments earlier or how solid I thought my commitment was, my flesh would scream and I'd cave in like a startled soufflé.

"Choose life." Again and again those words would come to me. I'd be faced with the temptation to forgo my food plan for the day or neglect the exercise I'd purposed to do and the words would come: "Choose life." I'd want to blow off a commitment I'd made or stay in bed instead of getting up early to invest in my relationship with the Lord, and His Word would come to me: "Choose life." On one occasion I heard a third-party report about someone and wanted to share the "news" (aka gossip), but the words "Choose life" echoed in my heart, calling me to make a godly choice.

To choose life is to choose God and His way of doing things. Can I choose to override the gentle nudge of the Holy Spirit bringing

God's Word to my remembrance? Yes. The still, small voice of the Lord doesn't come with a two-by-four to enforce compliance. Sometimes I've tried reasoning with the gentle voice, but the more time I've invested in reading, meditating on, and speaking the Word of God, the less I want to go against His guidance—thank God!

What is life? More importantly, *who* is Life? Jesus said in John 14:6, "I am the way, the truth, and the life." He also said that His words are spirit and life.[1]

"Choose life" is a loaded phrase, isn't it? I invite you to meditate on it for a moment right now and ask the Lord to reveal what it means for you personally. For example, it may mean turning away from unhealthy habits or desires and choosing to develop a new, healthier habit. It can mean purposing in your heart to say something positive when something negative is on the tip of your tongue. "Choose life" can be the cue you give yourself to change your behavior and go in another direction. Ask the Lord to guide you. In the space below, write the answers you sense Him speaking into your heart ("My sheep hear My voice").[2]

Lord, what does "choose life" mean for me personally?

How can I choose life in those areas of my life in which You want me to change?

Lord, remind me and help me choose life when I'm tempted to go in a direction that's displeasing to You. I want to walk in newness of life, following You, my Shepherd and Guide.

Freedom in the Narrow Way

Jesus said, "Enter by the narrow gate; for wide is the gate and broad is the way that leads to destruction, and there are many who go in by it. Because narrow is the gate and difficult is the way which leads to life, and there are few who find it."[3] The note in the margin of my Bible mentions that the Greek word for "difficult" can be translated "confined." There is liberty in the loving confines of God's narrow way, for "broad is the way that leads to destruction."

According to the world's definition, "freedom" is the ability to do whatever we want to do without limits or constraints. But freedom without self-control isn't really freedom at all; it's bondage to every whim of the flesh and every temptation of our adversary, the devil. The freedom God gives us in Christ is truly liberating.

Self-control can guide us on that liberating, narrow way. Why is the fruit of self-control so important? Also known as restraint or temperance, self-control protects us from the enemy like the thick stone walls of an ancient city protected it from invading forces. "Like a city whose walls are broken down is a man who lacks self-control."[4] But when our lives are fortified by the fruit of self-control, we experience real freedom and peace, like the inhabitants of a protected city.

Temptations will come—and not just the temptations to overeat or forgo exercise. Most of us are also tempted to give up standing by faith. If you're seeking to hold fast to God's promises in any area of your life, you may be tempted to quit many times. You can overcome that temptation by praying, speaking the Word of God aloud, and shouting, "I choose life!" You can also thank God in advance for the victory and sing praises to Him. Do whatever will stir your faith to *believe* and *take positive action* despite the circumstances that are screaming the opposite message at you. Our circumstances and feelings are temporary and subject to change. Truth, however, is eternal. And the Word of God is truth.

Simple Dietary Guidelines for Fat Loss and Energy Gain

Please remember that the most important part of your fitness plan is your spiritual fitness—your relationship with the Lord. Look to Him first to help you set sensible goals and follow a good food and exercise plan. Choose appropriate scriptures and write them on index cards to take with you or post in places where you'll see them often. Meditate on them. Memorize these "God thoughts" to renew your mind and become better acquainted with the true Source of your strength: the Lord.

Now, here are eight practical nutrition guidelines to help you on your Total Fitness journey.

BUSY WOMAN'S QUICK TIP
WHAT IS YOUR FOOD?

Jesus said something quite remarkable to His disciples in John 4:34: "My food is to do the will of Him who sent Me, and to finish His work." What an extraordinary thing to say! His "food" (a noun) became an action verb ("do").

Since we are Christians ("little Christs"), we're to be "imitators of God as dear children."[5] How many of us can say our food is to do the will of Him who sent us? I ask myself, "What am I really feeding on physically, mentally, and spiritually? Have I 'eaten' today? Have I been doing the will of the Father or merely filling my mouth and mind with 'empty calories'?"

I purpose to eat at the Lord's table, in His presence, so that His will may be done in my life. His food is truly filling and fulfilling. Have you "eaten" today?

---

1. If It's as White as Snow, Just Say No

In other words, just say no to white sugar...as well as high-fructose corn syrup, maltose, dextrose, lactose, and all the other little "oses." Sugar doesn't promote the growth of cells or lean muscle tissue, and it does nothing for your overall health. It does, however, make you fat.

Sugar in its various forms has lots of calories but no nutrients. It robs your body of vital nutrients so it can be processed. It can also lead to increased levels of insulin in the bloodstream. Insulin not only regulates blood sugar and helps transport vital nutrients to the cells, but it also sends the signal to your body to store fat. If you have elevated insulin levels, it's almost impossible to lose weight. So cut the sugar!

Look at the labels on the foods you buy. If sugar (in any of its forms) is among the first three or four ingredients listed, say, "No, thank you." Remember that fruit juices contain high amounts of fructose (fruit sugar), so if you're interested in losing fat, you'd be better off drinking pure water.

Say no to junk food and fat-free processed foods as well. The fats have been replaced with more sugar and processed carbohydrates, so steer clear of them.

Also say no to starchy carbohydrates, such as white flour (regular pasta, white bread, or any products made with white flour), white rice, and cornstarch. Foods made with these products convert from starch to sugar in your body—and, as we know, sugar turns to fat.

Cut back on white potatoes; eat them sparingly. Although potatoes have more nutritional value than white rice, they're still a starch that turns to sugar when they're metabolized.

Oh, by the way, although cauliflower is as white as snow, you don't have to say no to it. It's definitely our antioxidant-rich friend!

2. Include Lean Protein in Three Meals and Two Snacks

Lean muscles are what the busy woman needs to burn fat and have a fit, strong physique. Protein contains essential amino acids that are the building blocks of healthy, lean muscle tissue. Eat four servings of protein a day. That means including a lean-protein food in each of your meals (breakfast, lunch, and dinner) and at least one of your snacks, and preferably both. Good lean-protein meat sources include hormone-free chicken and turkey breast, lean grass-fed beef, and fish. Soy protein, nuts, eggs, low-fat dairy products (such as cottage cheese and other low-fat cheeses), and vegetable-protein products are also good nonmeat protein sources.

For snacks, choose a protein shake that is low in fat and has less than 5 grams of sugar and 5 grams of carbohydrates, such as Praise-Fast meal replacement Shakes (see Resources). If you prefer a protein meal-replacement bar, pick one that's at least one-third protein by weight (check the grams) and has less than 5 grams of sugar and no more than 10 grams of carbs. (Some have a lot of calories, sugar, fat, and carbs, so read the labels carefully.)

Instead of getting a canned protein drink at the supermarket, go to a health-food store and buy a protein powder that meets the same criteria as a protein bar. In your blender mix together 2 scoops of protein powder, a few frozen strawberries, a teaspoon of fiber, ice cubes, and 12 ounces of water for a thick, creamy shake.

BUSY WOMAN'S QUICK TIP
DITCH THE MICROWAVE?

Are we sacrificing more than quality for the convenience of having a microwave oven? Unfortunately, yes. Food cooked in a microwave loses much of its nutrition. One study showed that broccoli cooked in a microwave loses 74 to 97 percent of its flavonoid antioxidants, which help protect the body from cancer. By comparison, steamed broccoli lost only 11 percent or less of its antioxidants.[6] Some European studies have linked foods cooked in microwave ovens[7] to possible health risks that include hormonal imbalance and cancer.

After reviewing some of this information, my husband and I decided to ditch the microwave a few years ago. The only time we almost miss it is when we want to heat something up quickly, especially when we forget to take frozen food out of the freezer early! For us, the convenience isn't worth the apparent risks.

---

3. Leafy Greens, Cruciferous Vegetables, and Fruits Are Your Friends

We all need carbohydrates—essential carbohydrates from God's garden, not the carbohydrates found in processed starches and sugars. Fresh fruits and vegetables supply our bodies with vitamins and minerals and help provide essential fuel for healthy brain function. They also provide the fiber our bodies need. Scientists are continually finding disease-fighting phytonutrients and antioxidants in fresh fruits and vegetables. Have you noticed there haven't been similar scientific breakthroughs for Twinkies or chips?

People who eat diets rich in fresh fruits and vegetables are often able to reduce their blood pressure and tend to have lower levels of bad cholesterol. Numerous studies have shown that cancer prevention often hinges on the natural phytonutrients found in produce.

Green, leafy vegetables include dark salad greens (romaine, green- and red-leaf lettuce, Boston lettuce, and butter lettuce, but not iceberg lettuce), spinach, kale, parsley, and chard. Cruciferous ("cross-bearing") vegetables come from plants with leaves arranged in the shape of a cross. They include cauliflower, broccoli, arugula, cabbage, bok choy, collard and mustard greens, and Brussels sprouts. Other great green vegetables include snap peas, green beans, asparagus, and celery.

Good fruit choices include apples, grapefruit, strawberries, blueberries, lemons, kiwifruit, peaches, and plums. Although we consider them vegetables, avocados and tomatoes are actually fruits. Eat higher-glycemic fruits, such as bananas and dried fruits, sparingly. (For other nutritious vegetable and fruit choices, see the Nutritious Foods List in chapter 2.)

Corn, carrots, bananas, and watermelon have high starch or sugar content, so limit them if you're looking for greater fat loss.

We need to eat between 5 and 13 servings of fruit and vegetables daily (up from 5 to 9 servings just a couple of years ago). The USDA (U.S. Department of Agriculture) estimates that Americans are eating 20 percent more vegetables now than 35 years ago; however, the increase is mostly in potatoes—half of that amount is in french fries![8] It's no wonder the obesity rate has climbed so dramatically.

What is one serving of raw vegetables? It's equivalent to 1 cup of raw leafy vegetables or 1/2 cup of chopped raw vegetables. Here's another way of looking at it: A serving (one portion) of veggies is what you can fit in the palm of your hand—about the size of a deck of cards.

If you aren't eating raw vegetables at all, start with 1 cup. If you're already eating a cup or two, add another cup. (It's really a lot less than you think.)

An easy way to get a couple of servings of veggies in is to make a big raw-vegetable salad. Since dinner is the meal most families can eat together, have 1 to 2 cups of a simply prepared salad at each person's place setting. Typically, darker-colored vegetables have a higher nutrient content.

BUSY WOMAN'S QUICK TIP
MAKE YOUR OWN FRUIT-AND-VEGETABLE WASH

Combine 1 tablespoon of lemon juice, 1 tablespoon of baking soda, and 1 cup of water in a spray bottle. Keep this solution by the sink so you can spray all your produce before rinsing it under running water. Making your own veggie wash is easy and natural, and it costs just pennies.

---

4. Become a Fiber Fan

Fiber is important for more than regularity. We need to eat a minimum of 25 to 30 grams of fiber a day for good health. Fiber is essential for everything from proper digestion to disease prevention...and even weight loss. Once we're taking in the proper amounts of fiber and water, the colon (large intestine) starts moving more regularly (one to three bowel movements per day). Many people then begin losing those stubborn excess pounds, have more energy, and feel lighter. When the colon is functioning more efficiently, other body systems begin working better as well.

Fiber not only facilitates digestion, but it also slows the production of insulin and helps your body metabolize protein more efficiently. As fiber digests, it breaks down into acids that activate the fat-burning process.

Fruits and vegetables, such as apples and carrots (with the skins), are good sources of fiber, as are whole grains, lentils, and legumes (beans and peas). Another way to guarantee that you're getting a sufficient amount of fiber in your diet is to take a fiber supplement. You can mix a few teaspoons of psyllium-seed husks in water, juice, yogurt, or a protein smoothie. Freshly ground flaxseed meal sprinkled on salads or in juice is another option.

The more fiber you eat, the more water you need to drink because fiber and water work together to stimulate the colon. "Pasty" foods, such as pasta and white-flour products, can clog the colon, so eat sufficient amounts of fiber daily to help avoid hemorrhoids, irritable-bowel syndrome, and colon cancer.

BUSY WOMAN'S QUICK TIP
SWITCH SIGNALS

If you battle the temptation to eat when your body isn't hungry, here's something that's worked for a lot of people. Decide that the "I have to eat something" signal means "I'm going to exercise now" or "I'll see if the kids want to play a board game" or "I'm going to call, write to, or visit someone."

Are you tempted to eat when you are *avoiding* doing something? I sure am. Ask yourself, "What am I trying to avoid doing?" And then choose to do it. You don't have to be a slave to temptation!

---

5. Never Skip Meals

Since the beginning of time, food has been vital for human survival. God designed our bodies so if we don't eat sufficient quantities of food every few hours a starvation response kicks in, lowering our metabolism so that we burn fewer calories and hoarding fat to ensure survival. Sadly, in many countries today, famine and starvation are common. Unhappily, in most Western societies weight loss has become the primary goal.

Since hunger triggers the body's "starvation response," slowing down your fat-burning metabolism, if you skip meals or don't eat often enough, you sabotage your weight-loss efforts. The body will hold on to fat at all costs and *catabolize* (sounds like cannibalize, but it means "breaks down") its own muscles for fuel. That's one reason why severe calorie-restricted diets don't work. Results on the scale may look promising while you're dieting, but if your body is burning muscle instead of fat, it will quickly pile on fat after the diet (with less muscle to burn the fat than before). Many fad dieters have trained their bodies to become superefficient at hoarding fat. If this describes you, take heart—that vicious cycle can be reversed!

Just as you must put fuel in a wood-burning stove to get heat, you must fuel your body's furnace with food to burn fat. You must regularly eat enough of the right foods so your body doesn't perceive deprivation and trigger the starvation response. By eating "enough," I don't mean eating until you feel stuffed. Being *satisfied,* not stuffed, is the goal.

In order to lose weight, eat small amounts of food five to six times per day, every two or three hours. Have three well-balanced meals (breakfast, lunch, and an early dinner—not past 7:00) and two or three healthful snacks in-between. Have a lean source of protein with each meal and have vegetables with three or more of your meals. Supplement two meals with foods rich in fiber and have whole grains or legumes (beans or peas) at two of your meals.

If you really don't want to eat at some point during the day, it's okay to skip a snack, but *don't* skip a meal. To avoid triggering the starvation response, it's important that you don't go for more than three or four hours without something to eat. Sometimes you may be in a situation where it's inconvenient to eat or impossible to find something healthful to eat. At such times I've taken an amino-acids product, such as Catalyst by AdvoCare, to feed my muscles building blocks of protein and help prevent muscle breakdown.

BUSY WOMAN'S QUICK TIP
FAMILY MEALTIME FIGHTS EATING DISORDERS

If you have children, you can help them (especially your daughters) avoid developing an eating disorder by having sit-down family meals on a regular basis. A study by the University of Minnesota discovered that girls who ate meals with their families at least five times a week had a 75 percent lower incidence of unhealthy eating behaviors, such as abusing diet pills, purging, or chronic dieting to control their weight.[9] Boys who ate with their families also had a reduced risk of excessive dieting behaviors, although the effect was not as great.

One of the researchers, Dianne Neumark-Sztainer, a professor of epidemiology at the University of Minnesota, said, "Since society has so much influence on adolescents because of the high prevalence of obesity and the pressure to be skinny, many girls are turning to unhealthy ways of controlling their weight." She went on to say that "prioritizing structured family meals that take place in a positive environment can protect girls from destructive eating habits."[10]

If you're married and have a difficult time getting everyone together for the dinner hour because of busy schedules and activities, start a family tradition of eating breakfast together instead. Researchers said it didn't seem to matter which meal families had together. What made the biggest difference was that family meals took place on a regular basis. Prayer and fellowship around the table also make a big difference!

If you're single and are used to eating meals in front of the television, try eating at least one meal at the dinner table every day, Invite a friend over to eat with you once or twice a week. Turn that TV off! Many women who eat in front of the television inhale their food and don't keep good track of their caloric intake or their portion sizes. If eating at the dinner table alone doesn't sound appealing, create a welcoming atmosphere by playing music in the background or decorating the table with flowers or candles.

Since you'll be eating more often, it's also important to pay close attention to portion size. For fat loss and energy gain, you want to eat small- to moderate-sized meals.

6. Count Your Portions Instead of Counting Carbs or Calories

If you want to lose excess fat and you're eating all the right things (low-fat and low-sugar foods) at the right times (three meals and two snacks), perhaps your portion sizes are too large.

As mentioned, a serving (portion) of most foods is equivalent to what can fit into the palm of your hand. That's about the size of a deck of cards or 20 grams. If you don't have a food scale, I recommend purchasing one. It's an eye-opener to realize that portion sizes are a lot smaller than most of us imagine.

Each of your three regular meals should consist of three to five portions of food: one or two servings of protein, one or two servings of living food carbs (such as vegetables or fruit), and a serving of starchy carbs (such as whole grains and legumes, but no white-flour products). For weight loss, eat your complex carbs at breakfast and lunch so you have time to burn off the energy these food produce (so it won't wind up around your midsection, hips, and thighs). Add small amounts of good fats (olive oil, nuts, seeds, and essential fatty acid supplements such as flax or fish oil capsules) to round out your eating plan.

A balanced snack should include two portions of food, ideally including protein for building lean muscle mass.

7. Enjoy a "Free Day" Once a Week

If you're making good progress with your nutrition plan, allow yourself one "free" day to eat some of the foods you've been avoiding during the week. Don't go crazy, of course, but if you've been thinking about lasagna or pizza and haven't had any in a while, go ahead and have it on your day off. Just make sure that one day off doesn't turn into a second and a third. For most people, knowing they have one free day makes disciplining themselves the rest of the week doable. You'll also be eating so "clean" the rest of the week that what you eat on your day off shouldn't set you back. If, however, you haven't made the progress you wanted to make during the week, use your free day as a catch-up day.

In time you'll probably find you prefer lighter fare. You may discover that the foods you used to crave don't hold the same power over you and that *nothing tastes as good as being clean and lean feels.*

BUSY WOMAN'S QUICK TIP
AN EASY WAY TO COUNT PORTIONS

The following is a breakdown of recommended food portions for each meal and the snack you eat in a given day, as well as some examples. Remember, quality proteins come from foods such as eggs, meat, soy, seeds, nuts, and low-fat dairy products. Simple, good-for-you carbohydrates include fruits and vegetables, whole grains (but no white-flour products), and legumes (beans, peas, and lentils).

1. *Breakfast*—one protein portion, one living food-carb portion, one starchy-carb portion. Examples: one egg, half a grapefruit, and a slice of whole or sprouted grain toast with a serving of butter or almond butter, or whole grain cereal topped with sliced strawberries and low-fat soy, dairy, or almond milk.

2. *Midmorning snack*—one protein portion and one living food-carb portion. Examples: low-fat cottage cheese and an apple or a small handful of almonds and some tomato slices.

3. *Lunch*—one portion of protein, two living food-carb portions, and one starchy-carb portion. Examples: open-faced turkey sandwich on one slice of bread with a big veggie salad on the side or a soy burger on a whole-grain bun with a vegetable salad.

4. *Midafternoon snack*—one protein portion and one living food-carb portion. Examples: one tablespoon of almond butter on two celery stalks, or a protein shake with fresh or frozen strawberries.

5. *Dinner*—one or two protein portions and two living food-carb portions (optional: one starchy-carb portion). Examples: chicken with lots of steamed veggies (with an optional small portion of whole-grain pasta or brown rice) or tofu stir-fry with lots of veggies and a salad. (For weight loss, add another portion of living food carbs in place of the optional whole-grain starchy carb. You don't need the extra energy in the evening that these dense carbohydrates give you. Protein for body rebuilding and repair along with vegetables is the best combination.)

For more ideas, see the Nutritious Foods List in chapter 2. Experiment with different vegetables and whole grains. One whole-grain combination my family enjoys with lunch or dinner is short-grained brown rice and rye. It's an inexpensive and deliciously chewy mixture that's easy to make and can double as a tasty hot or cold breakfast cereal.

8. Have Your Dessert—and Eat It, Too

Try to fit your dessert into your portion count. How about low-fat yogurt (protein) with sliced fruit (living food carb)? Another low-fat dairy or soy-protein product with either a whole-grain starchy carb or a living food carb would work just as well, as would a protein smoothie. Use your imagination and think "portion size" instead of calories and carbs.

Here are some super dessert ideas (these could also double as a snack).

- a protein shake (soy, whey, or egg-white protein) with berries

- an apple or half a banana with 1 tablespoon of peanut butter or almond butter

- half a cup of low-fat frozen yogurt or ice cream with berries and 1 tablespoon of crushed almonds or walnuts

- sliced fresh fruit (1 cup) with a dollop of low-fat yogurt

- blueberries, strawberries, and raspberries (1-1/2 cups) layered in a glass dessert cup and topped with low-fat yogurt (sprinkle with stevia or 1 teaspoon agave nectar or honey)

"Garnish Your Plate with Praise"

Most of us are accustomed to thanking God for our meals before we start eating. In my book *BASIC Steps to Godly Fitness*, I proposed encircling our dining experience with praise—or what I call "garnishing your plate with praise."[11] Isaiah 55:2 quotes the LORD, "Listen carefully to Me, and eat what is good, and let your soul delight itself in [be satisfied with] abundance." Do you see the three parts of that scripture?

1. "Listen carefully to Me."

2. "Eat what is good."

3. "Let your soul [be satisfied with] abundance."

As we grow in our walk with the Lord, we realize that He is genuinely interested in everything that concerns us—even what we eat. By being willing to discipline our flesh, we become more sensitive to His leading.

One day as I was prayer journaling, I wrote, "Father, how can I best reach and maintain the healthy ideal weight and size for me?" The Lord led me to Isaiah 55:2 and this plan: Give the Lord a portion of your food every day. How? Since you can't physically give food to the Lord, substitute it with a portion of praise and thanksgiving. Your portion is what you eat; the portion you give to the Lord is your offering of praise and thanksgiving. The physical food you leave on your plate serves as a symbol of the sacrifice of praise you offer Him from your heart. Save the "food given" for another meal.

You know how full you feel when you completely throw yourself into praise and worship? Or if that's not your style, recall a time when you were so tremendously thankful for an answered prayer or the Lord's intervention at the exact moment you needed Him most that you thought you'd burst. That's what you want to accomplish!

I used to eat way past the point of satisfying my physical hunger to fill a void of a different kind. Have you? If you'll eat *slowly* enough to be sensitive to when your stomach is satisfied, you'll recognize when to stop eating—even if there's still a little food on your plate. Put down your fork, and if you're alone, start praising the Lord aloud. Thank Him for who He is in your life. Worship Him for His amazing attributes and His love for you. Have a time of sweet communion between the two of you. After all, He is the "bread of life" that truly satisfies.[12] You may be amazed at how quickly you feel satisfied.

When you're eating at home with your family or out at a restaurant and sense you're no longer hungry, put down your fork and silently praise and worship the Lord. Thank Him in your heart. You don't have to be showy about it. No need to be rude or hyper-spiritual and shut everyone else out because you're "communing with God." Another choice is to tell those at the table something wonderful the Lord has done for you or someone you know. In the psalms David often spoke of telling others about the Lord's marvelous works. That's praising God! No one has to know why you're sharing if you don't want them to. If you have kids, it's also a great opportunity to tell them why you love and trust the Lord. You might begin by saying, "I was thinking about how much the Lord loves us." You'll be giving glory to God ("garnishing your plate with praise"), satisfying your soul with abundance, and sharing God's love and provision at the same time!

Sweet 16 Weight-Loss Tips

Following these weight-loss tips can give your body the added boost it needs to burn fat and shed unwanted pounds.

1. *Keep cool.* The cooler your body stays, the more heat it has to produce to keep you warm, which burns more calories. Feeling a little on the cool side means you're also burning fat. Always keep as cool as possible when exercising.

2. *Eat slowly and stop when you're no longer hungry*—before you feel full. Be sensitive to the amount of food you're eating. Remember: A single portion of food (one serving) is about the size of a deck of cards.

3. *Instead of eating out, make your own meals* to take with you to work or when you go on outings. There are many hidden calories in restaurant food. As an extra benefit, you'll save money.

4. *Take a leisurely stroll* about 30 minutes after dinner. If you're married and have kids, make it a new family tradition. If you're single, invite someone along. Enjoy each other's company and walk at a gentle pace for 15 to 20 minutes to help your food digest. Don't walk briskly or jog because vigorous exercise interferes with digestion. A stroll will also help you keep from snacking after dinner.

5. *Drink a gallon of refrigerated, purified water or sparkling water each day.* Your body burns about 150 calories to heat 1 gallon of cold water to body temperature so it can be voided. Even though this is more than the recommended eight to ten 8-ounce glasses of water (64 ounces) a day, if you choose to drink up to a gallon of refrigerated water a day, you'll burn an extra 150 calories!

6. *Quickly drink a glass of cold water when you feel a cheat comin' on.* If you can, brush and floss your teeth as well. Meditate on a scripture (such as Ephesians 6:10—"I am strong in the Lord and in the power of His might!") and speak it aloud.

7. *Post positive notes and instructions around the house where you'll see them*—on the refrigerator, the bathroom mirror, your computer, and the front door. Use reminders like "Drink your water!" "Take your lunch!" "I will win!" "I choose life!" and "I can do all things through Christ who strengthens me!" These positive reminders are strong motivational tools to keep you focused and heading in the right direction.

8. *Get seven to nine hours of sleep each night.* Adequate sleep is essential for health and weight loss. Studies have shown that sleep deprivation can lead to weight gain.

9. *Do not skip meals, especially breakfast!* Skipping meals won't help you lose weight. The opposite is true. The body perceives deprivation as starvation and will hoard fat and consume muscle instead. Your body needs to feel satisfied and have proper amounts of nutrients available to shed fat and build muscle. Remember to eat starchy carbs (whole grains, legumes) during the day to give your body ample time to burn off the energy they produce so it won't be stored as fat.

10. *Read a book every week that is motivational in nature.* Feeding your mind and spirit is just as important as feeding your body.

11. *Avoid eating processed, low-fat and no-fat foods.* Eat from God's bounty (fruit, vegetables, lean-protein foods). Your body will perceive these as *real* foods and use them to help you lose fat.

12. *Choose high-fiber fruit* (such as berries or an apple) when you want something sweet. Fiber is an important part of your diet and speeds fat loss.

13. *Picture yourself as fit, healthy, and strong several times a day.* See yourself wearing a lovely outfit and feeling great while visiting friends, being on vacation in a beautiful setting, or playing with your children or grandchildren. As you make positive choices every day, you'll be one step closer to that stronger, healthier you!

14. *Avoid exercising too much.* Okay, who said, "Fat chance!"? Too much exercise can create hormonal imbalances, which can lead to muscle loss and excess fat storage. Actually we don't receive benefits from exercise *when* we're exercising. Our bodies experience the benefits during times of rest and recovery following exercise. If you're following a nutritious food plan (low fat and sugar), you won't need to burn off a lot of excess fat during exercise. You'll also save yourself and your joints the additional wear and tear.

15. *Engage in a craft or hobby in the evening* rather than mind-lessly watching television or surfing the Internet, which can lead to mindless snacking. Is there a hobby, skill, or language you've wanted to learn but haven't had the time to pursue? How about making Tuesday and Thursday evenings family game time—without snacks?

16. *Don't use the scale to measure your weight-loss progress.* Scales aren't an accurate gauge for weight loss or overall health. At the start of the Total Fitness program take your measurements with a tape measure and weigh yourself. Then put the scale in the closet for a few weeks. (Okay, at least for one week.) Chart your progress by realizing how much better you feel, checking to see how your clothes are becoming looser, and taking your measurements once a week. Every inch lost equals approximately 1-1/2 pounds of fat gone. Remember that you'll be building lean muscle at the same time, so while your clothes may feel looser, the scale may not reflect the lost weight because muscle weighs more than fat.

MAKING IT PERSONAL

1. God said in Deuteronomy 30:19, "I call heaven and earth as witnesses today against you, that I have set before you _____ and _____, blessing and cursing; therefore choose _____, that both you and your descendants may live."

2. I'll admit I haven't always made the best choices. I can start changing that now. Instead of _____ _____, I will choose life and _____. Instead of choosing to _____ as I have in the past, I will _____. With God's help, I can choose life!

3. Include lean protein in _____ meals and _____ snacks.

4. Examples of lean-protein meat sources include hormone-free _____, _____, and _____. Good nonmeat protein sources include _____, _____, _____, _____, and _____.

5. It's important that you don't go for more than _____ hours without something to eat to avoid triggering the starvation response.

6. Portion sizes are important. A portion is about the size of a _____ of _____.

7. Three things I can start doing right away from "The Busy Woman's Sweet 16 Weight-Loss Tips" are:

-

-

-

YOUR FITNESS PERSONALITY

*Personality is that peculiar, incalculable thing
that is meant when we speak of ourselves
as distinct from everyone else. Our
personality is always too big for us to grasp.*

OSWALD CHAMBERS
MY UTMOST FOR HIS HIGHEST

The busy woman doesn't have time to waste when it comes to getting fit. So how would you like to find the ideal way to manage your weight and increase your level of fitness based on your unique personality profile?

Your personality identifies you as an individual in the eyes of other people. Ole Hallesby wrote in his classic *Temperament and the Christian Faith*, "Everything has been created for God's kingdom. So too the temperaments. They are a part of the richly colored life which, when everything is fulfilled, will constitute the kingdom of God."

You are unique. There's no one exactly like you. Just as you have a God-given physical blueprint consisting of your DNA and heredity, you also have a God-given emotional blueprint consisting of your personality. Your personality not only sets you apart from others, it also serves as your very own set of colored glasses through which you see the world and the people around you.

My discussion of the four temperaments or personalities in this chapter is based on the marvelous work of Christian authors

Florence and Marita Littauer.[1] Their program—The Personalities—was founded on the teachings of the ancient Greek physician Hippocrates (yes, of the Hippocratic oath). The Personalities aren't pigeonholes into which everyone is to be neatly organized. Rather, a study of these four basic personality types can help us work from our strengths and fortify our weaknesses while better understanding the people around us. Have you noticed that not everyone acts and responds the same way you do? Since we can't change people (and we've tried, haven't we?), understanding them comes in very handy.

The Littauers' teaching on The Personalities has been credited with saving a number of marriages and has helped people understand how to relate to their children, siblings, and coworkers more effectively.

Understanding Your Personality Type

Could understanding your personality type help you find a health and fitness program more suited to your temperament? I believe it could. For example, if you don't enjoy being around a lot of people when you exercise, joining a gym and being part of a big kickboxing class probably wouldn't be for you. If you did decide to take a class like that as a challenge, after a few weeks you might begin finding other things more important or enjoyable to do than going to the gym. It could become another one of those self-improvement projects you began but didn't finish. Then you might be tempted to blame yourself or get down on yourself and ask, "Oh, what's the use?" But if you follow a program more suited to your personality, you'll probably enjoy yourself and be more likely to stick with the new routine.

Let's take a look at some of the strengths and weaknesses of the four personality types. First, take the following test to discover your primary and secondary temperaments. Put a check mark next to the character traits that best describe you. If you're not sure, ask someone who knows you well. When you're done, add up each column's check marks and write down the totals.

PERSONALITY TEST

A	B	C	D
__ loves excitement	__ aggressive	__ insightful	__ tolerant
__ humorous	__ goal oriented	__ considerate	__ content
__ spontaneous	__ independent	__ organized	__ relaxed
__ positive	__ confident	__ idealistic	__ good listener
__ friendly, outgoing	__ realistic	__ trustworthy	__ flexible
__ storyteller	__ bold leader	__ artistic/musical	__ peacemaker
__ unpredictable	__ impatient	__ timid	__ hesitant
__ loud voice	__ controlling	__ suspicious	__ sluggish
__ disorganized	__ insensitive	__ overly sensitive	__ plain vanilla
__ absentminded	__ blunt	__ self-doubting	__ indifferent
__ chatty	__ authoritarian	__ perfectionist	__ unenthusiastic
__ attention seeker	__ workaholic	__ loner	__ lazybones

____ *Total A*   ____ *Total B*   ____ *Total C*   ____ *Total D*

Which columns had the most number of check marks? Which had the second most marks? If most of your marks were in column A, your personality type is primarily Popular Sanguine; if B, Powerful Choleric; if C, Perfect Melancholy; if D, Peaceful Phlegmatic.

Here is a quick overview of the character traits of the four personality types.[2]

1. Popular Sanguine

Basic desire: have fun

Emotional needs: attention, affection, approval, acceptance

Controls by: charm

Communication style: open, expressive body language; loves to hug; laughs easily; speaks before thinking; can talk to anyone at any time

Slogan: "Are we having fun yet?"

Nicknames: the Talker, the Storyteller

Friends and work: makes friends easily; loves people; envied; never a dull moment; apologizes quickly; volunteers for jobs; starts in a flashy way; inspires and charms others to work

For stress relief: goes shopping; has a party; eats to cheer up and reward herself

Causes of depression: life is no fun; feeling unloved

Energy level: high energy level; frenetic pace; may have sudden spells of exhaustion; energized by people

Weaknesses (strengths carried to the extreme): exaggerating; losing sight of the truth (extremes of being talkative and a good storyteller)

Spiritual strengths: grace, joy

Scripture: "Rejoice in the Lord always. Again I will say, rejoice!" (Philippians 4:4).

2. Powerful Choleric

Basic desire: have control

Emotional needs: loyalty, sense of control, appreciation, credit for work

Controls by: threats of anger

Communication style: quick; bold; to the point; points or wags finger in your face; pounds fist; gives quick commands or orders; doesn't tolerate small talk; just the facts!

Slogan: "Just do it!"

Nicknames: the Doer, the Boss

Friends and work: has little need for friends; will lead and organize; is usually right; excels in emergencies; goal oriented; sees the whole picture; delegates work; thrives on opposition

For stress relief: works harder; exercises more; stays away from unyielding situations

Energy level: highest energy of all personality types; needs little rest; thrives on controlling people

Weaknesses (strengths carried to the extreme): workaholism; mercilessly drives others to succeed (extremes of being dynamic, active, and goal oriented)

Spiritual strengths: justification, diligence

Scripture: "By the grace of God I am what I am, and His grace toward me was not in vain; but I labored more abundantly than they all, yet not I, but the grace of God which was with me" (1 Corinthians 15:10).

3. Perfect Melancholy

Basic desire: have perfection

Emotional needs: sensitivity, support, space, silence

Controls by: threats of moodiness

Communication style: few gestures, little touch; precise, accurate; speaks when she thinks she can contribute; closed life; shares only with closest friends; thinks first, then speaks; good listener; shares on a self-determined need-to-know basis

Slogan: "If it's worth doing, it's worth doing right."

Nicknames: the Thinker, the Perfectionist

Friends and work: makes friends cautiously; faithful and devoted;

deep concern for others; moved to tears of compassion; can help solve problems; schedule oriented; high standards; detail conscious; orderly; finds creative solutions; likes charts, graphs, figures, and lists

For stress relief: withdraws from people; reads, studies, meditates, prays; goes to bed

Energy level: moderate energy; needs peace and quiet; drained by people

Weaknesses (strengths carried to the extreme): critical of others; skeptical of compliments (extremes of being analytical and meticulous)

Spiritual strengths: knowledge, wisdom

Scripture: "Be perfect, therefore, as your heavenly Father is perfect" (Matthew 5:48 NIV).

4. Peaceful Phlegmatic

Basic desire: have peace

Emotional needs: peace and quiet; feelings of worth; lack of stress; respect

Controls by: procrastination

Communication style: relaxed body language; calming presence during other's stressful times; speaks only when she has something of value to say; hesitant to offer opinions; uninvolved, almost fearful to get involved; soft voice; dry humor

Slogan: "I don't care. It doesn't matter."

Nicknames: the Watcher, the Relaxer

Friends and work: easy to get along with; pleasant and enjoyable; inoffensive; enjoys watching people; has compassion and concern for others; competent and steady; has administrative ability; avoids conflict; mediates problems; good under pressure; finds the easy way

For stress relief: turns on the television; eats and sleeps; tunes out people and circumstances

Energy level: lowest energy of all personality types; needs much rest; drained by people

Weaknesses (strengths carried to the extreme): avoids responsibility; becomes lazy (extremes of being easygoing and relaxed)

Spiritual strengths: acceptance, peace

Scripture: "Peace I leave with you. My peace I give to you" (John 14:27).

Overcoming Your Weaknesses

Can you see some of yourself and your loved ones in these thumbnail personality sketches? Perhaps you can better see why some fitness programs you've tried in the past didn't work for you.

As a shy, Melancholy/Choleric child, I found it almost impossible to enjoy sports and group games. Later, as a teenager, other young people often thought I was stuck up. I was painfully shy and would often walk on the other side of the street to avoid people. Onstage, however, was a different story. As a natural-born actor, I discovered that the stage was a platform where I could exert some control. I felt safe there—the first place I felt comfortable in a crowd. Audiences were predictable (when I could make them laugh!). But in everyday life, people weren't that predictable or eager to applaud. So when I was offstage, I retreated to the hollow comforts of food and alcohol to cope with the emotional pain and anxiety I felt.

Later, as a Christian, I discovered that my personality with its frustrating flaws also had useful strengths. Constant self-criticism stemmed from a desire for perfection that could be channeled into an aspiration to excel and be the best I could be. I turned to God to help me overcome my fear of people. The Bible taught me fear of people is a dangerous trap and trusting in the Lord will keep me safe.[3] The Word of God offered me hope that I could change—or rather, that I could be changed and transformed by the renewing of my mind, just as Romans 12:2 says.

We all have weaknesses. That's one of the reasons we need one another in the body of Christ. Our strengths shore up the weaknesses of others, and our insufficiencies can be balanced by the sufficiencies of our brothers and sisters. Thankfully, in the areas where we all are utterly hopeless, Christ is our all-sufficiency!

One of the benefits of becoming more aware of our personality weaknesses is that we can choose life and change. Let's not make excuses, such as "I can't help that I'm _____. After all, I'm a Sanguine [or Choleric, Melancholy, or Phlegmatic]." Having that attitude only gives us another reason why we don't want to change, and we know God takes no pleasure in our stubborn self-satisfaction and complacency.

For example, when I sense a fear of people coming on, I can either choose life by facing the fear head-on and leaning on the Lord as we walk through that momentary valley of the shadow of death together or I can choose to run away, retreating into my old, familiar prison. If I choose to run away, I have failed the test again, but God will give me opportunities to take that particular test many more times until I pass it. So in your weaknesses decide whether you want to be like the Israelites in the Old Testament and take 40 years to cross the desert or take the "Hallelujah Jumping Express." It's up to you.

Don't let your weaknesses become a flashing red light that stops you cold in your tracks. Instead, consider them a green light that keeps you moving through them or a yellow light to *yield* to the Lord and lean on His power to bring you safely to the other side.

BUSY WOMAN'S QUICK TIP
FITNESS TIPS THAT FIT YOUR PERSONALITY

It doesn't matter what form of exercise you choose as long as it's something you'll be motivated to do on a continual basis. The three parts of a great fitness program include (1) *aerobic activity* for cardio-vascular health, endurance, and fat metabolism (burning body fat); (2) *flexibility training* (stretching) for improved range of motion and joint health; and (3) *strength training* (resistance training) for building lean muscle, boosting metabolism, and strengthening bones. Here are some examples.

1. *Aerobic activity.* Low to moderate aerobic activities include walking, raking leaves, playing with your children and grandchildren, mowing the lawn, gentle rebounding on a mini-trampoline, and walking up a flight of stairs instead of taking the elevator. Higher-intensity aero-bic activities include an aerobic dance class (as well as spinning or kickboxing), aerobic dance to gospel music, brisk walking, brisk prayer walking, faster-paced rebounding on a mini-trampoline, tennis, rac-quetball, biking, rowing, running, jogging, skating, cross-country or downhill skiing, swimming, and using a StairMaster, treadmill, or sta-tionary bike.

2. *Flexibility training.* I suggest PraiseMoves or any other form of gentle static stretching (no ballistic or bouncing stretches), as well as ballet and other gentle-movement techniques that incorporate flexibility train-ing. My reasons for not suggesting yoga or tai chi are explained in chapter 9, "PraiseMoves—The Christian *Alternative* to Yoga." There are also a number of good books and DVDs that focus on the benefits of stretching—from pain management, rehabilitation, and preventing sports injuries to developing a graceful, lean, flexible body.[4]

3. *Strength training.* There are a number of ways to build strength, including participating in toning or body-sculpting classes, lifting weights (free weights or weight machines), and using resistance bands or your own body weight (such as push-ups, bent-knee sit-ups or abdominal curls, and chin-ups). I also suggest trying the Slow-Cadence

Exercise (SCE) presented in chapter 8, a Working Out with the Word (WOW) class or DVD, or the Gimme Ten Workout. (For more information on the WOW Workout and the Gimme Ten Workout, see the resources section at the end of the book.)

Designing Your Fitness Program

Let's consider your personality in planning the best fitness program for you. Quite frankly, if you try to follow a program that's radically counter to your temperament, you probably won't stick with it for any length of time, as long as you have a choice. This isn't army boot camp, after all.

There's no such thing as a Couch Potato Personality, either. Every personality type can be fit and healthy. Some of us may have to use a bit more spiritual dynamite to blast ourselves out of our droopy doldrums. Others will have to keep their tempers in check when the scale doesn't seem to budge or the splits don't come as easily as they did 20 years ago—if they ever came at all! We all can be in good shape.

The fitness programs described on the following pages have been designed with the needs and interests of each personality type in mind. Included is an exercise plan, a nutrition plan, and a list of things to avoid doing. One of the benefits of following the program that's designed for your personality type is that you'll be more likely to stick with it. As you do, you'll find your motivation growing and your fitness level improving day by day.

Fitness Program for Sanguines

If you're a Sanguine, your basic desire is to have fun. So this needs to be a key component in any fitness program designed for you. Without adding some spice to your workout, boredom can set in and you will quickly lose interest and motivation.

Exercise plan. Follow these guidelines for a fun and fulfilling workout:

- As you begin your workout, present your body to God as "a living sacrifice," as it says in Romans 12:1. Ask God for direction. Give your desires, concerns, plans, and goals to Him. Choose life.

- Choose a fun, fast-paced program at a gym or fitness center. Go for variety!

- Put an exercise class together at your church or home and invite your friends. Make it a party!

- Pick a friend to be your walking buddy or accountability partner. Encourage and motivate each other. (You are so good at that!)

- Plan your exercise times; write them on the calendar and follow through.

- If you find yourself getting bored, don't give up—just try a new routine.

Nutrition plan. As a Sanguine, you need to incorporate fun into your food plan as well. Try these suggestions:

- Follow a simple, sensible food plan you can maintain easily without having to follow a lot of rules (KISS = Keep It Simple, Sweetheart!).

- Select one "free" day a week when you can enjoy some of your fun foods without guilt.

- When planning social gatherings or outings with your friends, focus on fellowship and activities not related to food (such as going to a play or visiting a trendy dress shop).

- Pick a nonfood reward to give yourself when you reach specific goals. Set goals all along the way so you'll enjoy more rewards.

What to avoid. Your personality weaknesses can interfere with your fitness program. Write reminders for yourself and keep them handy in case you're tempted to give in to your weaknesses. For example:

- Don't expect immediate results; stick with your program. Change will happen!

- Don't go for a quick fix (such as a crash diet). Lasting results come from lifestyle change.

- Don't buy every cute exercise outfit or piece of new equipment you find. Save a new purchase as a reward when you achieve specific fitness goals.

Fitness Program for Cholerics

What Cholerics want most is a sense of control over their lives and environment, so this must be a key component in your fitness plan. Without a sense of control or a feeling that you're achieving your fitness goals, you may find yourself angry and frustrated, which will have a negative impact on your fitness program.

Exercise plan. Follow these guidelines for a challenging, goal-oriented workout:

- As you begin your workout, present your body to God as "a living sacrifice," as it says in Romans 12:1. Ask God for direction. Give your desires, concerns, plans, and goals to Him. Choose life.

- Be patient with yourself. "Imitate those who through faith and patience inherit the promises."[5]

- Select uncomplicated exercises (from an exercise class, a book, or DVD) that will produce proven results in the least amount of time.

- Find a personal trainer or exercise class that will challenge you.

- Keep track of your progress.

- You may do best with early morning exercise; get your workout done and out of the way early and shower just once.

Nutrition plan. As a Choleric, you need to incorporate structure and goals into your food plan to give you a sense of control. Try these suggestions:

- Follow a solid, sensible food plan you can maintain.

- No matter how busy you are, eat breakfast every day. Skipping meals is counterproductive.

- Cut back on caffeine and get more sleep. This helps with stress as well as weight loss.

- Set realistic, achievable goals . Write them down in your planner or put them on index cards. Use these cards as bookmarks or slip them into your wallet or checkbook where they're easily accessible.

What to avoid. Your personality weaknesses can interfere with your fitness program. Write reminders for yourself and keep them handy in case you're tempted to give in to your weaknesses. For example:

- Don't be a slave driver. You'll get better, long-lasting results and prevent burnout if you treat your body with respect and care.

- Don't skip meals. Your body will trigger the starvation response and begin storing fat.

- Don't opt for coffee instead of water. You need to stay well hydrated.

- Don't jump into exercising without warming up first. Stretch or gently run in place. Not warming up properly increases your risk of injury.

- Don't try to do too much too soon. Balance is the key.

Fitness Program for Melancholics

If you're a Melancholy, your basic desire is for perfection. The challenge in developing a fitness program designed for your personality type is to ensure that the focus is on progress and aiming for excellence rather than on perfection. Otherwise you may become discouraged and critical of yourself and lose motivation.

> *Exercise plan.* Follow these guidelines for a structured workout you can excel at:
>
> - As you begin your workout, present your body to God as "a living sacrifice," as it says in Romans 12:1. Ask God for direction. Give your desires, concerns, plans, and goals to Him. Choose life.
>
> - Aim for progress (growth), not perfection. Be patient with yourself! Lasting change takes time.
>
> - Use a comprehensive fitness program that has everything you need already in it. (For ideas see Resources.)
>
> - Schedule your workouts in your daily planner or calendar.
>
> - You may prefer working out at home to a DVD or a daily fitness program on TV rather than joining a big exercise class at a gym.
>
> - If you join a fitness center, ask to be guided through the best program for you (weight machines, classes, etc.). You may want to work with a personal trainer to perfect your program.
>
> - Work out to your favorite music for added inspiration and motivation.
>
> - Keep a journal and write down your feelings, prayers, goals, and successes.
>
> - Chart your progress as your fitness improves.

Nutrition plan. As a Melancholy, you need to incorporate structure into your food plan and aim for progress (growth) rather than perfection. Try these suggestions:

- Follow a solid, sensible food plan you can maintain.

- Decide that you'll take action *before* you have all the information. If you wait until you've analyzed everything and planned out every detail, you may never get started.

- Be patient with yourself! Remember: aim for progress, not perfection.

- Write down your daily food plan and commit it to the Lord every day.

- If you'd like to keep score, work toward getting as close to 100 percent each day as possible: 20 percent each for a sensible breakfast, lunch, and dinner; 10 percent for each of two snacks; and 20 percent for exercise. Rate how well you did each day, and go for a passing grade. (Remember that a "perfect" score isn't possible every day.)

- Decide on an appropriate nonfood reward to give yourself when you reach your first small goal. (Don't wait until you reach the finish line.)

What to avoid. Your personality weaknesses can interfere with your fitness program. Write reminders for yourself and keep them handy in case you're tempted to give in to your weaknesses. For example:

- Don't expect perfection of yourself. You'll learn as you go; this is a lifestyle change.

- Don't try to make a total lifestyle change overnight. Think progress, not perfection.

- Don't give in to discouragement or the temptation to criticize yourself or others if no one else wants to join you.

- Don't be rigid. Allow yourself to rest. Plan a day off into your schedule.

Fitness Program for Phlegmatics

What Phlegmatics desire most is peace, so this must be a key component in any fitness plan designed for you. Without a positive, easygoing environment that gives you a sense of peace and well-being, you may find yourself feeling stressed out and drained, which will work against your fitness goals.

> *Exercise plan.* Follow these guidelines for a positive, peace-focused workout experience that will fill you rather than drain you:
>
> - As you begin your workout, present your body to God as "a living sacrifice," as it says in Romans 12:1. Ask God for direction. Give your desires, concerns, plans, and goals to Him. Choose life.
>
> - Make small changes every day. You can build up to the next step one day at a time.
>
> - Find a fitness book or program that will guide you step by step.
>
> - Work with a friend or personal trainer who will motivate you and hold you accountable. Ask that person to help you assess your growth—how you've improved and where you may need to add a bit more effort to see greater results.
>
> - Plan your exercise times; write them on the calendar. Make an appointment with yourself and stick to it.
>
> - Increase your energy expenditure a little more every day. You don't have to be uncomfortable to become fit. Consider how you can add a little more movement into your day—starting now.
>
> - Congratulate yourself on each new step you've taken. Yes, it is a big deal! You're worth it.

Nutrition plan. As a Phlegmatic, you need a realistic food plan with reasonable goals. You also need to find ways to motivate yourself that don't add stress to your life or drain your energy. Try these suggestions:

- Follow a simple, sensible food plan you can maintain easily without having to follow a lot of rules (KISS = Keep It Simple, Sweetheart!).

- Make a list of what you need from the store and take it with you when you shop.

- Go for several small, simple upgrades in your food plan rather than trying to make major changes all at once.

- Plan meals and snacks *beforehand* instead of waiting until you're hungry.

What to avoid. Your personality weaknesses can interfere with your fitness program. Write reminders for yourself and keep them handy in case you're tempted to give in to your weaknesses. For example:

- Keep change manageable so you don't become overwhelmed. Don't worry about the details; just start where you are with what you have now. Remember: KISS = Keep It Simple, Sweetheart!

- Don't listen to the "Oh, what's the use?" monster. He's a liar.

- Don't wait until the first of the month or a Monday to begin making changes. You can take one small step today.

- Don't graze in front of the television or computer or while reading. Pay attention! Don't give in to the temptation to eat when you're involved in sedentary activities.

No matter what your personality type, you can be a "fit witness" for the Lord, incorporating fun, control, perfection, and peace into your daily routine—by His grace. *Rejoice!* God is in *control,* and He will keep you in "perfect peace" when your mind is stayed on Him![6]

MAKING IT PERSONAL

1. After taking the personality test, I discovered that I'm primarily _____ and secondarily _____.

2. Now that I know my personality type, I can see why I enjoy _____ so much, but I really don't like

_____.

3. Considering my personality type and the suggestions presented in the corresponding exercise plan, I'm going to try _____

_____

_____

and see how I like it.

4. Considering my personality type and the suggestions presented in the corresponding nutrition plan, I'm going to try _____

_____

_____

and see how I like it.

FITNESS FOR
THE BUSY WOMAN

*Bodily exercise profits a little, but
godliness is profitable for all things,
having promise of the life that now
is and of that which is to come.*

1 TIMOTHY 4:8

I'll admit it. Exercise isn't my most favorite activity. There, I said it. I have a love–hate relationship with exercise. I dislike it most before I do it, I tolerate it for the first few minutes, and then I start enjoying myself. By the end I'm feeling pretty good about myself, and I *love* the results.

As busy women, how can we incorporate physical activity into our already demanding lives? Just as we looked at how to make smart food choices more convenient, let's begin making some twenty-first-century conveniences "inconvenient" so we can see ourselves as active people instead of sedentary ones. For example: walk to destinations whenever possible, park farther away from the entrance at work or the store, and hide the television remote (with spousal agreement, of course!).

Are you like me? Do you find excuses for not exercising come easily? "I'm too busy!" "There's no time!" "It's boring!" It's tempting to give in to those excuses, but God is leading us to live more balanced lives. If we get too far off on one side of the road or the other, we'll fall into a ditch.

Some women have told me, "Hey, the Bible says that exercise

doesn't profit anything." Well, not quite. In his letter to Timothy, the apostle Paul recommended that Timothy train himself to be godly in character just as an athlete trains to be physically superior. Paul wrote, "Bodily exercise profits a little, but godliness is profitable for all things, having promise of the life that now is and of that which is to come."[1]

The Greeks of Paul's day held physical training in high esteem. Athletic events, such as the Olympics, were very important to them. Greek athletes were known and respected for their discipline and endurance, so it's not surprising that Paul sometimes used runners and races as metaphors for living the Christian life.[2]

In 1 Timothy 4:8, Paul says that although physical exercise may profit us for a little while during this life, it can't be compared with righteousness (right standing with God through Christ) and godliness, which benefit us here and eternally. People of the Bible weren't against physical exercise; it just wasn't a priority for them. They were active enough trying to keep food on the table and weight on their bodies. They definitely weren't concerned about keeping off pounds. In Bible times men and women lived arduous, physically taxing lives. Rarely do we see paintings of corpulent people unless they were members of the privileged aristocracy. It's not surprising then that our ancestors were able to eat large amounts of food and not become overweight. Their everyday lives were prolonged aerobic workouts. We, on the other hand, have to move our bodies not only to stay fit and healthy but also to keep from gaining excess weight. A 132-pound woman of today who works in an office setting burns about 720 calories of energy during an eight-hour workday. By comparison, our ancestors several thousand years ago burned 2,160 calories working and gathering food for their families over the same period of time.[3]

Present Your Body

Although exercise wasn't a priority in biblical times, Paul instructed believers to "present your bodies a living sacrifice."[4] He also counseled them to take care of their bodies, since they were "temple[s] of the Holy Spirit."[5]

Here's a sobering question: Do you think we'll be required to give an accounting to the Lord for the stewardship of our bodies and how well we've taken care of them during our lives? In 1 Corinthians 6:19-20 Paul wrote, "You are not your own...you were bought at a price" (the shed blood of Jesus Christ). Could that mean your body isn't yours but the Lord's? How well are you caring for His property?

The good news is that since your body belongs to the Lord, He has a vested interest in helping you care for it. Your body is not only the temple of His Holy Spirit; it's what you need to walk around this earth and spread the Good News that Jesus is Lord. The more fit and healthy you are, the greater probability you'll be around longer to carry out God's will for your life.

The enemy wants you to fail at your task—to fail horribly. Since you've accepted Christ, he knows you're going to heaven, but he certainly doesn't want you to help others get there. If your body is out of shape and lacking energy, it's difficult to do all the Lord is calling you to do. But you and the Lord working together can change that! "What?" you ask. "The Lord needs my help? But He's omnipotent, all-powerful, and in control!" Well, yes—and no. He is all-powerful, but He won't wrestle the cake fork out of your hand or pick up strings like a grand marionette Master and animate your body to take a brisk walk. You have to exercise your will to *choose* life and exercise.

Our Secret Weapon

As Christians we have a secret weapon against apathy and complacency when it comes to making changes in our lives. We have the weapon of the "sword of the Spirit...the word of God."[6] We can also sow any action we take as a seed to the Spirit that will reap lasting results, physically and spiritually. Whatever we sow "to the Spirit will of the Spirit reap everlasting life."[7] By sowing a seed of discipline in the area of fitness, for example, we can reap a healthy habit of regular exercise, a more active lifestyle, and the fit, trim body these habits yield.

Whatever we do "as to the Lord" brings supernatural help and increase because we're tapping into the heavenly realm for assistance. How can we make an exercise program a spiritual experience and receive heavenly help? Have you ever prayed while working out? No, I don't mean the "Lord, please help me!" prayer after 45 minutes into your step-aerobics routine. I'm talking about dedicating your exercise time to the Lord and asking Him to help you do your best and make exercise a healthy habit. How about presenting your body to God and praying, meditating on Scripture, or listening to gospel music while working out? What about communing with the Lord during a brisk walk or while exercising on the treadmill or stationary bike? Some of my friends use their morning walk as a time to pray for others. During the first part of their walk, they pray for our nation's leaders and the church and lift up the needs of their family and friends. On the way back home, they praise the Lord for answered prayer. If you and your friends are taking a walk, share something the Lord's done for you lately, pray, or encourage one another in the faith.

From a practical standpoint, it makes sense for busy women to combine spiritual and physical fitness—it's multitasking! Not only does it save time, but it's one way we can "pray without ceasing."[8]

All of these activities bring honor to God. My personal favorite (which is included on every exercise DVD we produce) is speaking and meditating on Scripture while working out. It's a great way to "transform your workouts into worship"!

Transforming Your Workouts into Worship

Is it possible to worship the Lord during a physical workout? Is that even a good thing to do? Does God honor such a practice? Let's talk about it. What is worship? According to the Bible, it's more than singing to God, as we do during praise-and-worship times at church.

In the fourth chapter of John, the Lord said to the Samaritan woman at the well, "God is Spirit, and those who worship Him must worship in spirit and truth."[9] What did He mean by "worship in spirit and truth"? Since the Bible needs no "private interpretation," the best thing to do is to let it interpret itself.[10]

If we understand what Jesus meant by "spirit and truth," we'll have a clearer picture of what He considers worship. He said in John 4:23, "The hour is coming, and now is, when the true worshipers will worship the Father in spirit and truth; for the Father is seeking such to worship Him."

How are "spirit" and "truth" described in the Bible?

After Jesus explained a hard-to-understand truth to His disciples in John 6, many disciples turned away. He said, "He who feeds on Me will live because of Me. This is the bread which came down from heaven."

"This is a hard saying," they said. "Who can understand it?"[11]

Jesus went on to explain that the words He spoke to them weren't ordinary words: "It is the Spirit who gives life...The words that I speak to you are spirit, and they are life."[12]

His words are spirit.

Later Jesus asked His Father to sanctify ("set apart for a holy purpose") the disciples and His subsequent followers by God's Word, saying, "Sanctify them by Your truth. Your word is truth."[13]

His words are truth.

Comparing these two verses, we see that the definitions of *spirit* and *truth* point to one thing: God's Word, the Bible.

Looking again at John 4:24—"God is Spirit, and those who worship Him must worship in spirit and truth"—we can assume that one way to worship God is through His Word, by reading it, meditating on it, speaking it aloud, and allowing our minds to be filled and saturated with it.

In PraiseMoves—my fitness book, DVD series, and alternative

to yoga—for example, we worship God as we meditate on, speak aloud, and allow our minds to be filled with and renewed by the Word of God. Is that okay? Well, what part of your life does the Lord *not* want to be part of? He wants to be involved in *every* area of your life, even during the time you devote to caring for your body, the Holy Spirit's temple.

In our hedonistic culture, many people seem to be consumed with (aka worship) the body. In contrast, let us be the sanctified ("set apart") ones who worship the Lord "in spirit and truth" in His Word. I invite *you* to transform your workouts into worship by incorporating the Word of God into your fitness program.

BUSY WOMAN'S QUICK TIP
THE PEDOMETER

A journey of 10,000 steps begins with one single step. A simple pedometer will help you keep track of the miles you walk as you go about your day. Walking 10,000 steps a day equals about five miles or 30 minutes of exercise. You can burn 2,000 to 3,500 extra calories a week this way. And what happens when 3,500 calories are burned? Right! One pound of fat disappears!

Since every 2,000 steps equal one mile, challenge yourself to increase your steps over a four-week period. Build up to 10,000 or more steps a day. Sitting at a computer all day makes that difficult, so it's important to schedule times to get up and move.

Wearing a pedometer during the day will be an eye-opener for some who think they walk all day but really don't. And those who think they don't do much by chasing kids around the house may be surprised to see how many steps they take throughout the day.

Note: Continuous aerobic activity for at least 20 minutes is important for cardiovascular health and is different from the start-and-stop walking around we do during the day. Four thousand steps (two miles) walked continuously over a 30-minute period has more aerobic benefit than the same number of steps walked over a 16-hour period.[14]

Fitting Fitness into Your Busy Day

Some great times for busy women to exercise are before a meal or one to two hours after a meal, although the *ideal* time to exercise is any time you'll do it and stick to it. Many women find that exercising first thing in the morning is best because they get it out of the way early and reap the benefits of a boosted metabolism all day.

Are there other times you can fit in a quick workout during your busy day? Yes! Did you know that the average American spends three hours a week on the telephone? That's not including telephone time spent at work. Imagine if you used only half that time doing some stretching and strengthening exercises. That's an extra 90 minutes of flexibility and resistance training per week!

If you work outside the home and you sit for long periods of time throughout the day, get up and move every 30 minutes or so to stave off mental fatigue and lethargy and for your overall health as well. Stretching and some type of movement every 30 minutes or so helps prevent repetitive stress injuries (RSIs).

The following exercises are designed to do just that—and more!

When exercising it's important to not overdo. If an exercise causes pain (not just mild discomfort), don't continue to do it. If you have physical problems, be careful to modify or avoid the exercises that might aggravate your condition.

QuickFits™—Speedy Exercises for Home, Office, and Travel

Even if you only have a minute of free time during your day, there's time to squeeze in one of the QuickFits exercises. As the name implies, they're quick enough to fit in just about anywhere. For an added spiritual workout, softly speak or meditate on the scriptural affirmation that accompanies each of the QuickFits exercises. Some of these you can even do while riding on airplanes, buses, and trains.

As I mentioned earlier, don't sit longer than 30 minutes at a time. If you're staring at a computer screen, stand and look into the distance. As long as no one is looking, roll your eyes and raise your eyebrows. Open and close your mouth as if silently saying, "Ahhh–ohhh." Reach your arms up and stretch as tall as you can. Before sitting down, get a glass of water.

Fitting in the following ten exercises during your day can help prevent repetitive stress injuries, such as carpal tunnel syndrome or pain in the fingers, hands, forearms, elbows, shoulders, neck, and back caused by repetitive movements (which are often experienced at computer stations).

1. Shoulder Rolls—For Relaxation and Good Posture

Scriptural affirmation: I will humble myself under the mighty hand of God that He may exalt me in due time; I will roll all my care over onto Him, because He cares for me (1 Peter 5:6-7).

Exercise: First, sit with your back straight and your arms at your sides. Inhale deeply into your abdomen as you slowly lift your shoulders up toward your ears and squeeze. Exhale as you lower your shoulders. Do this 3 times.

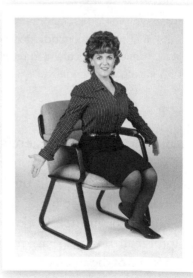

Next, sit on the edge of your chair, arms at your sides. Sit up straight, lifting up through the crown of your head as if trying to make yourself an inch taller. Your chin should be parallel to the ground and your feet flat on the floor. Take a deep breath into your abdomen as you roll your shoulders forward. Exhale as you then roll them backward, palms facing outward, toward the walls. Reach your thumbs back. Repeat 3 times. Keep your shoulders, neck, and face relaxed.

On the third repetition, keep your shoulders rolled back but bring your hands to your lap, palms up. This is perfect posture. Practice keeping your shoulders rolled back like this throughout the day (but after rolling your shoulders back, return your palms to normal position). Be aware of how much better your neck, back, and shoulders feel when they aren't slumped over a computer, sink, or shopping cart.

2. Gentle Neck Stretches

Scriptural affirmation: I will keep sound wisdom and discretion so they will be life to my soul and grace to my neck. I will walk safely in my way, and my foot will not stumble (Proverbs 3:21-23).

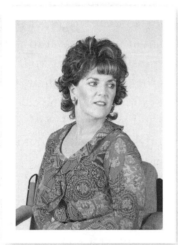

Exercise: While sitting (or standing), inhale, then exhale as you turn your head to look over your right shoulder. Inhale, then exhale as you return your head to front and center. Repeat on the other side and continue for 3 complete sets. The ideal is a 90-degree turn so your chin is positioned directly over your shoulder.

Next, exhale, bringing your right ear down to your shoulder. Gently place your right hand on the side of your head and stretch your left arm downward to increase the stretch.

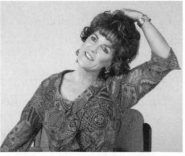

Breathe gently. Repeat on the other side, then return to center and slowly lower your chin to your chest. End the stretch by bringing your head back to neutral position.

3. Biceps Strengthener

Scriptural affirmation: I will gird myself with strength and strengthen my arms (Proverbs 31:17).

Exercise: Use a chair arm, desk, or table to do this exercise to tone the biceps (the front muscle in your upper arm). If using a desk or table, keep your back straight, with the small of your back pressed against the chair and your abdomen tight. If using a chair arm, turn as far to the side as possible, bringing your knees to the side of the chair. Check first to make sure the chair arm or desktop is stable so it doesn't go flying across the room when you lift up on it.

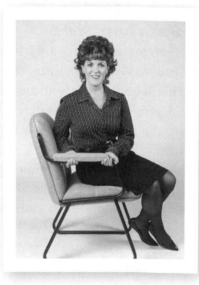

Now, reach under the desktop or chair arm, and keeping your arms at a 90-degree angle, press your elbows into your sides and press up with your hands (palms facing up). You should feel a contraction in the biceps. Hold for a count of 10, breathing gently. Relax for a moment, then repeat 2 more times. Keep your shoulders, neck, and face relaxed.

4. Hand and Wrist Exercises

Scripture: "Blessed be the LORD my Rock, who trains my hands for war, and my fingers for battle" (Psalm 144:1).

Exercise: First, put your hands at your sides and shake them vigorously for 5 to 10 seconds. Then with your arms out in front of you, palms up and elbows straight, gently press your fingers down and back with your opposite hand. You should feel the muscles of your inner forearm stretching. Breathe gently. Shake your hands.

Next, stretch your fingers apart as far as you can. Slowly rotate your hands from the wrists several times, first clockwise, then counterclockwise. Shake your hands one more time.

5. Turn-Away Twist in a Chair

Scripture: "Turn away my eyes from looking at worthless things, and revive me in Your way" (Psalm 119:37).

Note: This posture involves twisting your back, so you should take particular care not to twist too far or you risk aggravating any existing back condition. This should be a gentle stretch. Twist only as far as is comfortable.

While meditating on the scripture, you'll be *physically* turning your body away from your desk or computer while *figuratively* turning away from the worthless things of this world. (I'm certainly not saying your work is a worthless thing, though!)

Exercise: Sit up straight in your chair, keeping your feet planted firmly on the floor and the backs of your thighs pressed into your chair. Keep your abdomen tight and your pelvis tucked under to protect your lower back. Exhale and lift your torso as you gently turn to the right. Let your hands help you turn by holding on to the arm or back of your chair. Follow the twist with your eyes as you turn, and try to look over your right shoulder. Breathe gently as you hold the twist and consider this exercise's scripture.

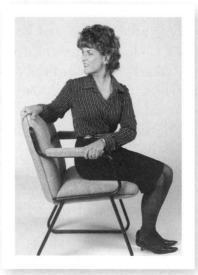

Inhale, then exhale as you come back to front and center. Repeat on the other side.

6. The Easy Yoke

Scripture: "[Jesus said,] 'Come to Me, all you who labor and are heavy laden, and I will give you rest. Take My yoke upon you and learn from Me, for I am gentle and lowly in heart, and you will find rest for your souls. For My yoke is easy and My burden is light'" (Matthew 11:28-30).

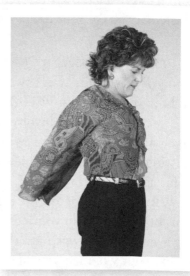

Exercise: First, stand and reach behind you, clasping both hands (palms facing each other) and interlacing your fingers. Take a deep breath, then stretch and straighten your arms as you exhale. Keep your chin down, pelvis tucked under, and body erect (abdominals tight) as you lift your hands toward the ceiling, breathing gently for 10 to 15 seconds. Relax and repeat.

Next, with your left hand gently pull your right arm across your body and reach your right hand over the opposite shoulder while pushing your right elbow against your left hand. Keep your head facing forward. Breathe gently. Hold a few seconds. Repeat on the other side. Do 3 sets.

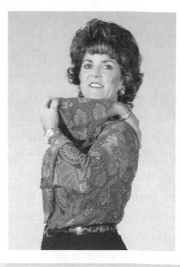

7. The Rainbow

Scriptural affirmation: When I see the rainbow in the clouds, I remember the everlasting covenant between God and every living creature. I remember the many mighty promises of God (Genesis 9:16).

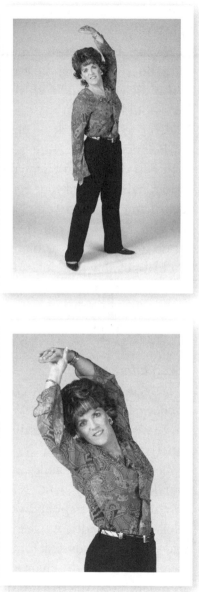

Exercise: This is a Praise-Moves posture. Stand with your feet shoulder width apart. Inhale, raising one arm (with your palm up) and bringing it over your head like a rainbow, ending with your palm facing down. Exhale and bend slightly to one side, feeling the stretch along your side. Let your opposite hand rest on one leg. Keep your pelvis tucked under and your abdominals tight to protect your lower back. Breathe gently and relax.

For more of a challenge, bring your opposite hand up to grasp the wrist of the overhead arm. Don't lean too far over to the side. Lift up instead. Continue to breathe gently. Don't hold your breath. Repeat on the other side.

8. Calf Raises

Scriptural affirmation: The LORD God is my strength; He will make my feet as swift and sure as a deer's, and He will help me

walk along high places (Habak-
kuk 3:19).

Exercise: If convenient, remove
your shoes to get the most out
of this exercise. Stand with your
feet shoulder width apart and
hold on to your desk or chair
for balance. (Make sure your
chair isn't on rollers.) Keep your
abdominals tight and your pelvis
tucked under. With your back
straight, exhale as you slowly
lift up onto your toes as high as
you can possibly go. Hold for a

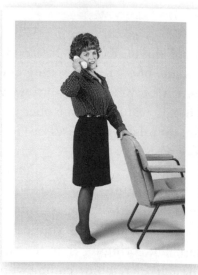

count of 3, then slowly lower as you inhale. Work up to a count of
20, breathing gently throughout. When you're stronger, balance on
one foot, placing your other foot behind the opposite calf.

9. Leg Lifts

Scriptural affirmation: Because I wait on the LORD, my strength
is renewed. I will mount up with wings like an eagle. I will run and
not be weary. I will walk and not
faint (Isaiah 40:31).

Exercise: Stand on one leg with
your knee slightly bent. Keep
your abdominals tight and your
pelvis tucked under. As needed,
hold on to a chair or desk for balance. (Make sure the chair isn't
on rollers.) On the exhale, lift
your opposite leg to the side with
the leg either straight or bent at a
90-degree angle. Breathe gently
as you hold this posture for a few

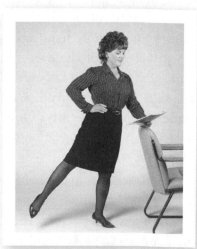

seconds, then lower your leg. Repeat until your muscle fatigues. Switch legs and repeat on the other side. You can add resistance by pushing against the leg you're raising.

10. Lunges

Scripture: "I press toward the goal for the prize of the upward call of God in Christ Jesus" (Philippians 3:14).

Note: This posture may aggravate any existing knee conditions. Use extreme caution and maintain proper form, ensuring that your knee is always aligned with your ankle and never moves beyond it. If necessary, you can modify the lunge by lowering your body less than 90 degrees.

Exercise: Stand with your feet slightly apart. Use a desk, table, or stationary chair (without wheels) for support. Tighten your abdominals and tuck your pelvis under. Take a giant step forward with one foot, inhale, and slowly lower your body until your front knee is at a 90-degree angle to the floor. It's *very* important to keep your knee in line with your ankle bone to prevent injury. Exhale as you slowly push yourself up with that leg until your knee is straight (but not locked). Lower and raise yourself several times and then return to the starting position. Repeat on

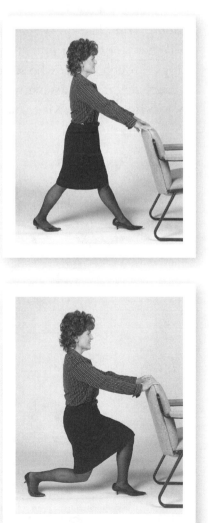

the other side. Alternate back and forth several times. As your fitness level grows, you'll be able to do more of these.

Higher-Powered QuickFits

For those of you who not only want to make the most of one minute but also want more of a physical challenge, I'm including a couple of exercises you can do to "pump up the volume."

1. Jump Thrusts

Perhaps the best scripture to go with Jump Thrusts is "I can do all things through Christ who strengthens me!" (Philippians 4:13).

Exercise: Start in a squatting position with your hands on the floor in front of you. Kick your feet back to push-up position and

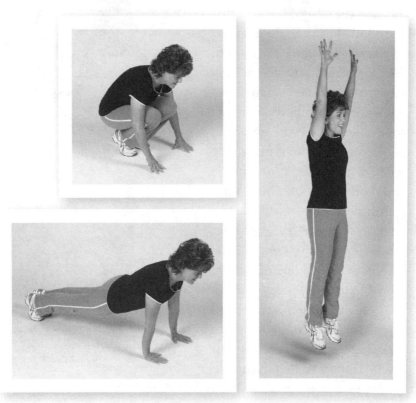

then immediately return your feet to a squatting position. Next, with gusto, leap as high into the air as you can. Repeat, moving as quickly as possible for 1 minute.

2. Mountain Movers

Mountain Movers are great for conditioning and increasing the body's core strength and endurance. During this exercise, meditate on Mark 11:23 (or shout it aloud!): "I say to the mountain, 'Be removed and be cast into the sea.' I do not doubt in my heart, but I believe the things I say will be done and that I will have whatever I say."

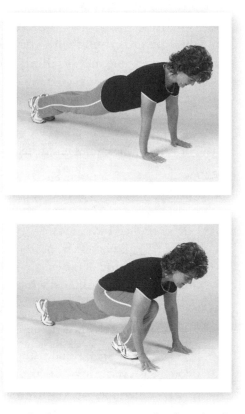

Exercise: Start in a push-up position with your legs extended. Keep your head in line with your body and your abdominal muscles tight throughout the exercise. Bring your right knee to your chest, with your foot touching the floor. Quickly bring it back to the starting position. Just as you're bringing your right foot back, bring your left knee to your chest. Alternate legs back and forth for 1 minute.

QuickFits in Flight

In addition to the neck and shoulder exercises described in the previous section, here are six exercises you can do to keep fit in flight (or while riding on a bus or train). Scriptures to focus on while doing QuickFits in Flight? How about 1 Corinthians chapter 13, the love chapter? Since God calls us to walk in love, these are excellent scriptures to memorize.

You can also claim the qualities of love for yourself by personalizing verses 4-8 in the following passage taken from the Amplified Bible. Fill in your name wherever you see a blank space (that's where the word "love" appears in the original) or simply say "I." Either way you'll be identifying with the most powerful force in all creation—the awesome, never-failing love of God!

_____ endures long and is patient and kind; _____ never is envious nor boils over with jealousy; is not boastful or vainglorious; does not display [herself] haughtily.

_____ is not conceited (arrogant and inflated with pride); _____ is not rude (unmannerly) and does not act unbecomingly. _____ does not insist on [her] own rights or [her] own way, for _____ is not self-seeking; _____ is not touchy or fretful or resentful; _____ takes no account of the evil done to [her][_____ pays no attention to a suffered wrong].

_____ does not rejoice at injustice and unrighteousness, but rejoices when right and truth prevail.

_____ bears up under anything and everything that comes, is ever ready to believe the best of every person, _____'s hopes are fadeless under all circumstances, and _____ endures everything [without weakening].

_____ never fails. [Amen!]

1. Biceps Strengthener

Raise one arm in front of you until your upper arm and elbow are straight in line with your shoulder joint. Relax your hand and tense your bicep as hard as you can. Hold for a few seconds and relax. Do as many repetitions as you can on each side, breathing gently. Do not hold your breath.

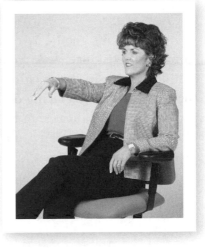

2. Triceps Toner

Sit on the edge of your chair and lean forward slightly, keeping your back straight. Bend your elbows, pressing them into your sides, and make fists. Exhale as you lower and straighten your arms, pressing your fists back and tightening the triceps muscles on the back side of your upper arms. Hold for a count of 10 to 20, breathing gently. Relax and repeat several times. This exercise works best if no one is sitting right next to you.

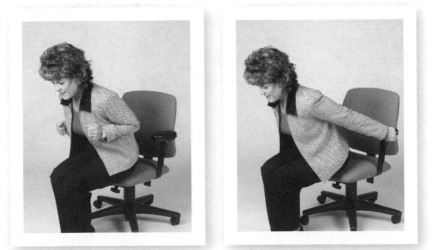

3. Chest Press

An oldie but goodie is the isometric (resistance) hold you can do by pressing your palms together with elbows facing out for a count of 20. Breathe in for a count of 10 and out for a count of 10. Repeat several times.

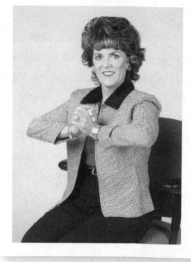

4. Seated Waist Trimmer

Reach up and grasp your elbows with both hands, keeping your head straight (neutral position) and your abdominals tight. Inhale deeply. Exhale as you lift up your torso and bend over to one side. Hold the stretch, breathing gently, then exhale as you return to center. Repeat on the other side.

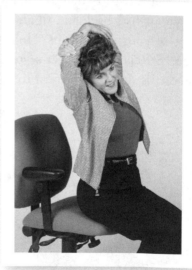

5. Leg Toner

Can you tone your thighs in flight? Sure! A great exercise for the adductors (inner thighs) is to make a fist with each hand and place them together between your knees. Exhale as you squeeze your knees together as tightly as you can while you add resistance by pushing out with your fists. Breathe gently while doing this isometric hold. Relax your face; don't hold your breath. Keep abdominals tight.

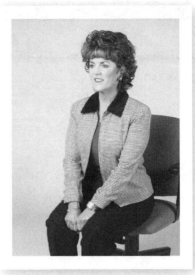

6. Tummy Tuck

Sit up straight and exhale all the air out of your lungs. Now, instead of inhaling, pull in your abdominal muscles as far and as high as you can. Hold for a moment, relax, and quickly repeat. Do as many repetitions as you comfortably can without breathing. Do this exercise before eating or 1 to 2 hours after eating (for obvious reasons!).

MAKING IT PERSONAL

1. These are the excuses I've always used when I don't feel like exercising: _____

   _____

   _____ .

2. Instead of giving excuses *not* to exercise, I'm going to change my mind and think of at least three reasons why it's important for me to be active. I want to exercise because _____

   _____

   _____

   _____ .

3. There are a lot of quick, simple exercises I can fit into my day. This week I'm going to try several from this chapter. In fact, I can do them right now! These are the three I'm going to do: _____, _____, and _____ .

4. One way I can transform my workouts into worship is to _____

   _____

   _____ .

BREATHING—ESCAPE
THE SHALLOWS

*The Spirit of God has made me, and
the breath of the Almighty gives me life.*

JOB 33:4

Oxygen is the most vital nutrient for our survival. We can go for weeks without food, days without water, but only a few minutes without oxygen. As Elizabeth Barrett Browning once wrote, "He lives most life whoever breathes most air." Unfortunately most of us are shallow upper-chest breathers who breathe in only enough air to barely fill the upper part of our lungs.

At the doctor's office, when asked to take a deep breath, most people's upper chest expands and their shoulders come up around their ears. Babies and young children are "belly breathers," meaning they naturally fill the lower part of their lungs with air. Singers, actors, and professional speakers are usually taught deep, diaphragmatic breathing for better vocal projection. I relearned how to be a belly breather in my early twenties at acting school. Athletes and those interested in fitness, stress relief, and overcoming anxiety also learn this type of breathing for better performance and relaxation.

Do you know which type of breather you are? Try this experiment. Sit up straight and put your hand on your abdomen. Now breathe in. Did your abdomen go in or out? If your abdomen went in on the inhale, you're only filling the upper part of your lungs.

If your belly relaxed and expanded on the inhale, you're breathing "from the diaphragm," as voice teachers say.

The diaphragm is a dome-shaped muscular wall between the rib cage and the abdomen. When we breathe deeply, the diaphragm moves down toward the abdomen, helping our lungs expand more fully. If you've seen drawings of the lungs, you may have noticed that they're larger at the bottom than at the top. Deep diaphragmatic breathing allows more oxygen to be taken in and more carbon dioxide to be released with each inhale and exhale.

At some point during childhood most of us switched from relaxed diaphragmatic breathing to shallower, more stressful chest breathing. Short, shallow breaths are one of the ways our bodies respond to fear and stress. This response is part of what endocrinologist Hans Selye called the "fight-or-flight syndrome." In our society pressures involving time, family, finances, health, work, and even traffic are commonplace so fight-or-flight responses take their toll. If we lived several thousand years ago, this fight-or-flight syndrome would have enabled us to respond quickly to danger. Shallow chest breathing would have prepared us to run from a predator or fight a hostile enemy. This type of breathing creates tension, whereas taking gentle, deep breaths brings relaxation.

If these quick, shallow breaths are the norm for you, you may be breathing too fast most of the time and also holding your breath in stressful situations. Upper-chest breathing requires more breaths per minute than abdominal breathing. Your heart is forced to work harder, your blood pressure rises, and your metabolism slows down, making weight loss more difficult.

If you're accustomed to shallow breathing, you may be operating at only a fraction of your lung capacity by filling only one-quarter to one-fifth of your lungs with oxygen. Since your lungs are designed to remove toxins, any stale air remaining in them may leave toxins behind, slowing your body down even more. Although the average pair of lungs can hold between 1 and 2 gallons of air, most people take in no more than 1 or 2 pints with each breath. If you aren't breathing sufficient amounts of oxygen, your cells aren't receiving the fuel they need to produce energy, burn fat, increase metabolism, bring mental clarity, and get rid of toxins. The result? Low energy, low metabolism, mental fatigue, and weight gain.

Learning to Inhale

Learning to breathe from your diaphragm takes a little practice if you're used to upper-chest breathing, but you can do it! Sit comfortably straight in a chair and loosen any tight or restrictive clothing. Place one hand on your abdomen just above your navel. Place your other hand on your upper chest just below your collar bone. Inhale deeply through your nose and try to gently make the hand on your abdomen move. You want your belly to expand like a balloon with air. Relax your abdomen. Your upper hand should move only slightly on the deepest part of the inhalation, gently filling the upper part of your lungs with air *after* the lower part is filled. Exhale gently through your nose. This is considered a complete, deep, diaphragmatic breath.

Don't worry if you don't catch on right away. Just keep at it.

Here's another way to learn natural diaphragmatic breathing. Lie down on a bed or the floor and place a book on your abdomen. As you inhale, make the book rise with each inhale. In drama classes, progressively heavier books were added to strengthen our ability to breathe from the diaphragm.

After doing either of these exercises a few times, close your eyes and relax even more. Try breathing in for a count of 4, hold for a count of 2, and then exhale to a count of 4. Become aware of any tension in your body and focus on gently releasing it.

There's nothing weird or New Agey about relaxing our bodies. I was concerned about that shortly after becoming a Christian. Some of the yoga practices I had learned involved deep relaxation techniques that I now know invite demonic activity. "Astral projection" (traveling outside the body) and breathing in certain "energies" (a technique called *pranayama*) were two things I did that gave place to the enemy in my life. As Christians, we have the Holy Spirit living within us, so we can't become possessed by demonic forces, but we can become *oppressed* by them. Believe me, dabbling in the occult is scary stuff. God even calls it "an abomination."[1]

Disciplining Our Bodies

The apostle Paul said, "I discipline my body and bring it into subjection, lest, when I have preached to others, I myself should become disqualified."[2] Eating right, exercising, and taking control of the flesh are all ways we discipline our bodies. We can also discipline them by helping them relax and operate more efficiently.

After practicing correct breathing for a while, you'll probably find yourself starting to breathe this way naturally. Again, some of the benefits of diaphragmatic breathing include:

- increased energy
- reduced mental and physical fatigue
- potential relief from long-term respiratory difficulties, such as asthma and bronchitis
- more efficient elimination of toxins
- improved blood circulation
- increased supply of oxygen and nutrients to cells throughout the body
- increased oxygen to the brain, aiding relaxation and mental clarity
- increased endurance
- a clearer, more radiant complexion
- improved, sounder sleep (Gentle, deep breathing helps your body relax.)
- relief from tension
- potential relief from depression (Since shallow breathers

are more prone to depression, deep breathing can offer relief.)

- potential relief from menopause-related hot flashes (according to some studies)

- increased flexibility (During stretching postures, such as found in PraiseMoves, deep breathing helps to gently stretch connective tissue, thus increasing flexibility. Postures are held for 3 to 5 breaths, with each breath taking approximately 10 seconds.)

- partial compensation for lack of exercise during recovery from an illness or injury

- increased control over the munchies (Instead of eating that unplanned snack, take 10 complete breaths. The desire to eat often passes.)

Over the years I've taught drama students diaphragmatic breathing and have received reports of increased relaxation, clearer thinking, better performance on tests, and relief from stage fright.

Deep breathing can be done anywhere. Instead of tensing up because of the long line at the supermarket, practice breathing techniques. People probably won't notice what you're doing, and they may marvel at your stunning sense of calm.

Breathing Exercises

I recommend staying away from any breathing exercises that advocate harsh, forceful inhalation or exhalation. These are common in the yogic *pranayama* breathing technique designed to "elevate consciousness." "Higher consciousness" is a carrot the enemy places before the gullible (as I once was) to deceive them into following his ways. It may seem appealing, but that tempting morsel is wrapped around a poison designed by the enemy, who comes "to steal, and to kill, and to destroy."[3]

Steer clear of techniques that advocate saying words you don't understand. *Mantras* are repetitive Hindu words associated with demonic spiritual activity. They might be low, melodic, mind-numbing sounds or harsh, explosive sounds. These sounds aren't harmless; they have a specific purpose. Don't call for the devil by saying words tied to demonic activity.

As Christians, "we have the mind of Christ,"[4] so any elevation of consciousness we try to force through physical means is not of God. There is no higher mind available anywhere than the mind of Christ! Use your breath to praise the Lord, as Psalm 150:6 encourages us to do: "Let everything that has breath praise the LORD"! Sometimes I've been known to exhale a relaxing, joyous "hallelujah" or "amen" at the end of a breath (but not repetitively). Jesus warned against the mindless repetition of words "as the heathen do."[5]

If you're taking acting or singing lessons, that's a different matter. I was often told to say silly things or to make funny noises to loosen up and train my voice. "Peter Piper picked a peck of pickled peppers" is nothing to be feared (unless, of course, you're *Mrs.* Peter Piper, because a peck of pickled peppers is a lot of peppers to prepare!).

I advocate breathing techniques that are purely for physical benefit and relaxation purposes. God gave you your breath. In Genesis 2:7 we see that God breathed life into Adam. God's breath enabled Adam to have a spirit. It's what transformed the dust of the earth into a living, breathing spirit-man made in the image of God.

As you do the following exercises, make sure you're breathing into the lower part of your lungs first. As a reminder, keep one hand on your abdomen when you start. Loosen any tight clothing that may keep you from breathing deeply.

The Easy-Does-It Breath. You may do this exercise standing, sitting, or lying down.

1. Inhale deeply to a slow count of 3.
2. Gently hold your breath to a count of 3.
3. Exhale slowly to a count of 3.
4. Repeat 3 or 4 times.

5. When this feels comfortable, increase each step by one (e.g., inhale to count of 4, hold for 4, and exhale to a count of 4).

The Three-in-One Breath. Father, Son, and Holy Spirit—our God, the Holy Trinity, is three in one. Contemplate this marvelous truth during this breathing exercise.

Opera singers and athletes may take in as much as 17 pints of air with one breath, while shallow breathers take in only 1 to 3 pints. With practice, you can increase your lung capacity with this exercise. Let's do it!

1. Stand up straight and stay relaxed. (This exercise may also be done sitting or lying down.) Loosen any tight clothing that may inhibit deep breathing.

2. Take a slow, deep breath for a count of 3: 1-2-3.

3. Gently hold your breath for a count of 12: 1-2-3-4-5-6-7-8-9-10-11-12.

4. Gently exhale for a count of 6: 1-2-3-4-5-6.

5. Repeat.

You're holding your breath 4 times longer than the inhalation, and the exhalation is twice as long as the inhalation. This ratio (1:4:2) remains constant. Make sure you're breathing into your abdomen first, and then allowing your rib cage to expand and your chest to rise slightly. Holding your breath extends the time for your lungs to exchange oxygen for carbon dioxide, allowing your blood to become more oxygenated.

When the count becomes comfortable, gradually increase the number of inhalations, holds, and exhalations, using the same 1:4:2 ratio: 4-16-8, then 5-20-10. If it's easier for you, start with 2-8-4. Remember to be gentle with yourself. You're coaxing your body to breathe more fully. It's not a forceful procedure.

As you become more conscious of your breathing and learn to

relax your body by breathing from your diaphragm, you may notice that situations that used to tie your stomach up in knots, tighten your neck muscles, and turn your shoulders into earrings no longer disturb you as they once did. You can now take in gentle, deep breaths and fully cast your cares on the Lord, telling your body to relax and your soul to "hope in God."[6]

If you've been involved in breathing practices that are based on yogic philosophy (such as the *pranayama* breathing technique I described earlier), and you feel a check in your spirit or a convicting tug at your heart, ask for God's forgiveness right now. Please don't wait until later. If you're unsure how to begin, this prayer can be used as a guide.

> Heavenly Father, Your Word says in 1 John 1:9 that if I confess my sins to You, You are faithful and just to forgive me of my sins and cleanse me from all unrighteousness. Father, right now I confess _____
> _____, and I ask You to forgive me as You said You would. I repent of this sin. I turn away from it, and I'm turning completely to You. Please wash me clean. Cleanse me from all unrighteousness. I receive complete cleansing this very moment from You in spirit, soul, and body—from the top of my head to the soles of my feet. Thank You for giving me a brand-new start! I refuse to look back; instead, I look forward and walk on in victory with You. I pray this in Jesus' name. Amen.

MAKING IT PERSONAL

1. _____ is the most vital nutrient for our survival. We can go for weeks without _____, days without _____, but only a few minutes without _____.

2. The benefits of deep breathing include _____
   _____
   _____.

3. I found the breathing exercises _____ (easy or difficult) to do.

4. To improve my breathing (or challenge myself more), I commit to do the following exercise(s) for the next few weeks:
   _____
   _____.

5. I will incorporate these breathing exercises into this part of my day: _____
   _____.

20 MINUTES TO BE FIT FOR THE KING

*She girds herself with strength [spiritual,
mental, and physical fitness for her God-given
task] and makes her arms strong and firm.*

PROVERBS 31:17 AMP
(brackets in original)

While most of us recognize the importance and benefits of exercise, the busy woman still runs up against a time crunch. So how much physical activity do we need to maintain good health? According to the 1996 *Surgeon General's Report* and the 2005 *Dietary Guidelines for Americans,* adults can receive general health benefits from doing at least 30 minutes of moderate-intensity activity (such as brisk walking) "most days of the week."[1] For many people, this would mean burning around 150 to 200 calories per exercise session.

According to a study in the *American Journal of Clinical Nutrition,* "Although 30 minutes of daily moderate-intensity physical activity may result in significant improvements in health, it appears that progressing to at least 60 minutes of physical activity may be necessary for enhancing long-term weight loss outcomes."[2]

I can hear some of you saying, "Sixty minutes of exercise a day! That's crazy! How can I possibly do that and have a life?"

Well, it gets even more interesting. The 2005 *Dietary Guidelines for Americans* recommends 60 to 90 minutes of daily, moderate-intensity activity "to sustain weight loss for previously overweight people."[3] Thankfully, not all studies had this high of a goal. A study conducted between 1999 and 2002 found that 30 minutes of moderate-intensity activity (the equivalent of walking 12 miles per week or 2.5 miles five days a week) was an adequate amount of exercise to prevent weight gain.[4]

What if your only physical activity is running errands, and your resistance activities amount to pushing away that second helping of chow? Good news! You can start where you are. How about 20 minutes of moderate-intensity activity several times a week? If you sleep 8 hours a night and are awake 16 hours a day, your waking hours can be divided into 48 20-minute segments. If you choose one of those 20-minute segments several times a week and dedicate it to the fitness of your "temple," you'll be in relatively good shape (literally and figuratively speaking!).

Sowing Seeds for an Abundant Harvest

In chapter 1, we discussed yielding to the fruit of the Spirit, such as when you decide to forgive a loved one instead of holding a grudge or punishing him (or her) by giving the silent treatment. When you forgive, you're yielding to the fruit of love that the Holy Spirit is developing inside you. When the person standing in line in front of you at the bank or grocery store is taking an interminably long time, you can decide to yield to peace and patience instead of clearing your throat, tapping your foot, and shouting.

If you have your Bible with you, I invite you to turn to the fifth chapter of Galatians. There is so much "meat" in this chapter, but let's look again at the fruit of the Spirit listed in verses 22 and 23: "love, joy, peace, patience, kindness, goodness, faithfulness, gentleness, and self-control." As busy women, we want something that will work for us not just some of the time but all of the time, every time. That's why I believe the Lord continues to bring us back to His Word over and over again. His Word to us is guaranteed to work every single time we believe it and apply it.

Earlier we discussed that lasting change in our physical and emotional natures won't happen as a result of a diet or exercise regimen alone, but from allowing the Holy Spirit to develop His fruit in our lives—especially the fruit of faithfulness, patience, and self-control.

The Holy Spirit is the Source of this fruit; He is the One who produces it in our lives. But we have a part to play in its development. Are there ways we can plant or sow seeds of faithfulness, patience, and self-control in order to experience lasting change in our bodies, minds, and emotions? Yes, I believe there are. Instead of just going through the outward motions of eating the right foods, drinking sufficient amounts of water, and getting daily exercise, let's consider how we can access spiritual help to change us on the inside at the same time.

Fruit Always Starts with a Seed

We can strengthen the fruit of the Spirit in our lives by choosing to yield to it on more occasions until it becomes second nature to us. For example, let's say you've chosen to yield to love so many times where children are concerned that if a friend's child misbehaves, you wouldn't have a fit. Love has become a way of life for you because you actively yielded to the Holy Spirit in this area so often. In fact, love is now part of who you are. This doesn't mean you won't succumb to temptation in this area ever again. But you have discovered that yielding to the Holy Spirit is the right and best thing to do.

But what if a particular fruit of the Spirit isn't first, second, or even third nature to you yet? That's where the biblical principle of sowing seeds can help. The Bible tells us that "while the earth remains, seedtime and harvest...shall not cease."[5] Everything in creation starts with a seed of some kind. Nothing great ever started large and powerful. In God's economy, things start small and grow. Perhaps that's why God said, "Do not despise these small beginnings, for the LORD rejoices to see the work begin."[6]

Can we plant seeds of faithfulness, patience, and self-control? Yes! This is another way we can strengthen the fruit of the Spirit in our lives. Interestingly, the process of sowing and reaping is discussed in Galatians 6, the chapter that immediately follows the passage about the fruit of the Spirit. Take a look at verses 7-8:

> Do not be deceived, God is not mocked; for whatever a man sows, that he will also reap. For he who sows to his flesh will of the flesh reap corruption, but he who sows to the Spirit will of the Spirit reap everlasting life.

At one time in my life, I sowed a lot of bad choices to my flesh and reaped the consequences, but then I learned about sowing to the Spirit. We can sow seeds of the fruit of the Spirit to the Lord and receive the life of the Spirit to help that seed grow and become part of our very nature. How? Let's look at this using the habit of drinking more water as an example.

Sowing in Action

We've read that drinking eight to ten 8-ounce glasses of pure water every day is good for us. Our human nature may say, "I hate water. I want Diet Coke." But instead of yielding to the flesh in this instance, we sow seeds to develop the fruit of...

- faithfulness by drinking more water every day
- patience by realizing it takes time to develop a taste for water
- self-control by choosing water over Diet Coke on a more consistent basis

This is how I began to develop a taste for water over soft drinks and other beverages. I'd wake up in the morning and say, "Lord, I'm going to drink eight glasses of water today. I want to be a fit witness for You. I want to develop the discipline to take better care of myself, and drinking water is part of that discipline." When I got water, I would hold the glass up to the Lord and say, "Lord, I'm doing this as unto You. I'm sowing this to the Spirit, and I ask that You help me make this a new, healthy habit in my life."

As I consistently dedicated these little actions to the Lord, sowed these little seeds on a regular basis to Him, God caused those seeds to take on life and grow. Suddenly I found myself *wanting* water instead of Diet Coke. Me, the six-pack-a-day girl! The same thing happened with exercise and making healthier food choices.

You can also use this principle when your flesh is screaming for an extra portion of food or a sugary snack or an extra 30 minutes of sleep instead of getting up to invest time in your relationship with the Lord. You can say, "I'm giving this up right now to plant a seed of self-control. I'm giving this to You, Lord."

God's Abundant Harvest

You've probably heard the expression "You can't outgive God." When you give, dedicate, and surrender something to Him, you always receive something greater in return. Can you imagine enjoying things you know are good for you but are hard to do now? If exercising regularly is something you have difficulty doing, choose one activity today or tomorrow and dedicate it to the Lord *first*. Plant a seed to the Spirit of God, and ask Him to help you develop the faithfulness, patience, and self-control to exercise on a regular basis so you can be a more fit witness for Him. Then take action. Go for that walk or swim and thank the Lord during that time for His faithfulness to you. Thankfulness and praise water the new seed you've planted.

I believe that as you do this on a consistent basis, you'll find your habits changing for the better. You'll begin to develop the fruit of the Spirit in areas of your life where you've been weak.

Yes, you'll be tempted by your flesh to go the other way...and sometimes you won't make the best decisions. (We're all human, and we haven't received our glorified bodies yet, so don't expect perfection!) But every time you yield to the Holy Spirit and "choose life," His fruit in you matures.

Faithfulness, patience, and self-control will gradually become second nature to you. And the fruit of the Spirit will grow in other areas of your life as well. Soon you'll be able to help others learn how to trust the Lord and follow these simple biblical principles of sowing and reaping!

Muscle—Yes! Fat—No!

Sadly, our bodies lose muscle mass as we age, and unless we're doing regular resistance (strength) training and eating properly, the rate at which this happens will increase. The average person between the ages of 25 and 55 gains 1 pound of fat and loses 1/2 pound of muscle every year. That means that by age 55, the average person will be 30 pounds heavier and carry 45 more pounds of fat!

As we lose muscle, our metabolism slows, we burn fewer calories, and we gain fat. Some of you may have noticed that even if you weigh close to what you weighed earlier in life, you're wearing larger clothing sizes. Let's say a woman lost 10 pounds of muscle and gained 10 pounds of fat between the ages of 30 and 40. She may get on the scale and see she weighs the same as she did ten years earlier, but her dresses are two sizes larger than they were back then. Why is that? Muscle is denser than fat. It takes up a lot less room. Five pounds of fat take up more than twice the space of 5 pounds of muscle. That's why a woman who does regular resistance training may weigh 130 pounds and wear a size 4 dress, while a nonathletic woman weighing 130 pounds might wear a size 10 dress. The women may weigh the same, but one woman's body has more compact, lean muscle compared to the other.

After the age of 50, most people are losing 1 percent of muscle mass each year, and many buy into the cliché "I'm no spring chicken. I guess I'm just getting old. I can't do what I used to do anymore." Happily, the Bible encourages us with these words: "Moses was one hundred and twenty years old when he died. His eyes were not dim nor his natural vigor diminished."[7] And Psalm 103 says, "Bless the LORD, O my soul...Who satisfies your mouth with good things, so that your youth is renewed like the eagle's."[8]

Physical strength is a by-product of muscle mass. The more lean muscle you have, the stronger you are. And the stronger you are, the better you feel. Your muscles are more able to do their jobs, thus indirectly improving the health of other systems in your body. Your liver functions more efficiently, feeding the muscles the nutrients they need. Oxygen is extracted from your blood more easily by the muscles, putting less strain on the pulmonary system (your heart and lungs). Your body becomes leaner, stronger, and healthier. What a blessing!

Although our bodies inevitably lose strength and muscle mass as we age, we can take some practical steps to mitigate these losses through strength training. And like Moses, we can trust God to help us maintain our "natural vigor"—our strength, vitality, and dynamism! We will experience significant benefits from building up our muscles regardless of our ages.

Now let's look at one exercise format you can "plant" in order to reap benefits for your spirit, soul, and body.

Slow-Cadence Exercise™—A Fitness Phenomenon

How would you like to exercise just once or twice a week for 20 minutes and get as much (or greater) benefit from it as you would if you were going to the gym five days a week? That can happen with Slow-Cadence Exercise (SCE)—resistance training done at a very, very slow tempo until your muscles fail.[9] Momentary muscle *failure* means your body *cannot* do more repetitions and maintain proper form, no matter what you tell it to do. This isn't the same thing as muscle *fatigue*, which means your body can still do one more rep even if it's screaming that it doesn't want to.

SCE is one way many people are restoring and maintaining their strength. Despite the benefits of traditional strength training, most people don't have the time to devote hours every week at the gym lifting weights. Besides, the constant strain of lifting the standard 3 sets of 8 to 12 reps per exercise can cause repetitive stress injuries to joints and tendons.

Unlike standard strength or resistance training, SCE doesn't depend on gravity or momentum. For maximum results you must perform each exercise as slowly as possible, using correct form, until your muscles momentarily fail. The good news is that because you're moving at such a slow pace, your muscles are forced to work harder so more can be accomplished in less time. Even though SCE may sound easy, it's not. It requires concentration and discipline but takes a very minimal amount of time.

SCE is based on the principle that removing momentum from an exercise forces the muscle to do all the work. Since the muscle is never able to rest, fatigue comes more quickly. When a muscle is brought to failure during strength training, tiny tears occur, creating blood flow to the site, which helps build the muscle.

The Slow-Cadence Exercise Workout

Before beginning this or any other exercise program, please see your doctor for a good overall checkup. This is pure wisdom. Know any physical limitations ahead of time. That way you can pay closer attention to building up those areas. You can also pray about them. The Lord will give you wisdom if you ask Him.

You can perform SCE at home or on the road. A variety of exercises can be performed with or without additional equipment, so if you're traveling and don't have access to your free weights or exercise ball, you can still have a very good and efficient workout.

When exercising it's important to not overdo. If an exercise causes pain (not just mild discomfort), don't continue to do it. If you have physical problems, be careful to modify or avoid the exercises that might aggravate your condition.

Equipment Needed

To get the most out of your SCE workout, you'll need:

- *An exercise ball.* An inexpensive, inflatable workout ball will come in handy for several of the SCE exercises. I've found it's also a lot of fun to use while sitting at the computer! Being "on the ball" helps you maintain the proper form, and you are more apt to hold in your stomach on an exercise ball than when you sit in a chair hunched over the computer. If you don't have an exercise ball, a sturdy stool will suffice.

- *Hand weights.* If strength training is new to you, I recommend starting with relatively light weights, such as 1, 2, or 3 pounds. If you've been training for a while, use the weights that suit you best. You can usually tell what the best weight is for you by doing 12 regularly paced repetitions of a bicep curl holding each weight. If you don't feel any difference after 12 reps, try the next heaviest weight. If the weight you use fatigues your muscle too quickly and it's hard to raise the weight one more time, try a lighter weight. You should feel as if you've done something, but not too much or too little.

  If you don't have a set of hand weights yet, you can use soup cans or gallon water jugs. Each cup of water weighs slightly more than 1/2 pound, so 6 cups of water in a gallon jug equals around 4 pounds. Okay, it's not glamorous, but it will do until you get those hot-pink hand weights you've had your eye on in the sports store!

- *Ankle weights.* These will come in handy for the leg raises. If you want to save some money, you could strap soup cans to your ankles, but quite frankly I think that's going a tad too far. Think how goofy you'd feel if a friend stopped by for a visit or your kids brought some of their friends over!

- *Exercise mat.* This will be useful for some of the floor work, and you'll also find it comes in handy for your PraiseMoves workouts. Mats are relatively inexpensive, but you can certainly use a thick towel until you can get one.

- *Towel* (optional). If your knees are sensitive, you may want to use a towel under them when you do push-ups. You can also use one under your hips for side leg raises.

Exercise Guidelines

Follow these four guidelines for each exercise:

1. Slowly and evenly count to 8 as you perform the first part of each exercise. Squeeze your muscles or hold at the top of the movement, then slowly lower to a count of 8.

2. In the beginning, it may be helpful to count one one thousand, two one thousand, three one thousand, and so on (or one Mississippi, two Mississippi…) until you're comfortable with the slow pace.

3. Once you have the timing down and feel you're moving at a slow and comfortable pace, add the scripture that accompanies each exercise. Say it aloud, under your breath, or meditate on it. Don't worry if you become distracted trying to do the exercise correctly. In time you'll be able to incorporate the Word into your workouts more effectively.

4. Do each exercise for approximately 2 minutes or to muscle failure.

Safety Tips

As you perform the SCE workout, it's very important that you keep these safety tips in mind:

- Don't hold your breath. Breathe as directed for each exercise—slowly and evenly, into the abdomen as much as possible.

- Don't scrunch up your face. Stay relaxed.

- Keep your cool. Have a fan blowing on you, and dress in cool, comfortable clothing—nothing too warm, tight, or restricting. This is one time you *don't* want to sweat. Let this be your no-sweat workout.

- If you feel pain, stop! Never say "No pain, no gain." Instead say "No pain, no pain—please, no pain!" (There's a definite difference between pain and discomfort. Pain is like an alarm going off in your brain telling you something is wrong. Discomfort is more like your muscles complaining because they'd rather take it easy. Pay attention to pain and push through discomfort.)

- Make sure you understand each exercise and the way it is to be performed before you begin. Read the instructions thoroughly. Don't assume that just because the photo looks like an exercise you've done before it is the same exercise. It most likely is not. Slow-Cadence Exercise is definitely different.

- You'll be doing each exercise for approximately 2 minutes or to momentary muscle *failure* (not muscle fatigue). Remember, muscle fatigue means your body is crying, "No more! I don't want to do anymore," but you could still do more if you told it, "I don't care what you say. Do more." Muscle *failure* means your body cannot do more repetitions and keep proper form, no matter what you tell it to do.

Slow-Cadence Exercises

The following exercises comprise every 20-minute SCE workout. You'll be amazed at the long-term benefits you experience from such a small investment of your time.

1. *One-arm pull-ups.* Use a 3-, 5-, or 8-pound hand weight for this exercise. Place your right hand on a stool or the back of a chair

without wheels for support. Your left arm should hang down at your side while holding a hand weight. Make sure to keep your left arm slightly bent; don't straighten it out or let the weight drag it down. Bring your right leg forward and bend it so your knee is in line with your anklebone. Keep your left leg extended straight behind you, and press your heel into the floor. Keep your head relaxed in a neutral position. Tighten your abdominals and tuck your pelvis under.

Lift the weight in your left hand very slowly to a count of 8, bending your elbow and aiming it out and up toward the ceiling while bringing the weight up to your chest and underarm. Breathe gently and evenly throughout the lift. Don't hold your breath! Keep your face relaxed and a fan blowing on you to keep cool.

When you get to the top of the lift, squeeze your arm and back muscles to a count of 2. Lower the weight just as slowly back to the starting position to a count of 8. Make sure to keep your arm slightly bent at the bottom of the lift.

At the bottom of the lift, immediately bring your arm up again to a superslow count of 8. Continue to keep proper form for 2 to 3 minutes or until momentary muscle failure. Repeat on the other side.

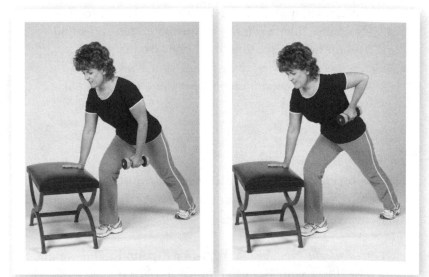

Scripture to meditate on: "He teaches my hands to make war, so that my arms can bend a bow of bronze" (Psalm 18:34).

2. *Bicep curls.* Use 3 to 5-pound hand weights. Sit up straight on a stool or on the edge of a sturdy chair, with a free weight in each hand. Keep your head in neutral position and your abdominals tight. Pull your elbows into your sides and slowly raise the weights toward your shoulders to a count of 8. Keep your upper arms and elbows pressed into your sides.

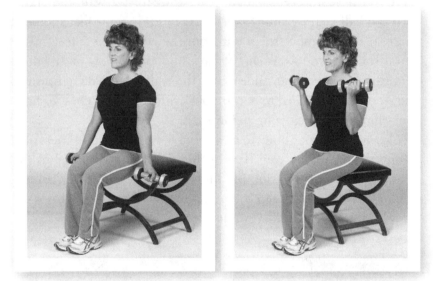

Breathe evenly throughout the lift; don't hold your breath. Bring the weights almost all the way up to your shoulders, curling your wrists in. Stop just short of the top and squeeze your biceps for 2 beats.

Slowly lower the weights, uncurling your wrists, to a count of 8. Keep breathing evenly. Pause at the bottom of the lift without straightening your arms, and immediately begin the slow-lift phase again to the measured count of 8.

Continue for 2 minutes or until muscle failure.

Scripture to meditate on: "Bear one another's burdens, and so fulfill the law of Christ. For if anyone thinks himself to be something, when he is nothing, he deceives himself...For each one shall bear his own load" (Galatians 6:2-3,5).

3. *Wall slide with exercise ball.* This exercise requires an exercise ball. If you don't have one, you can still benefit by sliding down a wall until your thighs are parallel with the floor. Hold the posture as long as you can. Then slide down to sit on a stool or on pillows placed below you.

If you have an exercise ball, place it against a wall and stand with the ball against your lower back. Position your feet shoulder width apart and move them out from the wall about 2 feet. Wear tennis shoes so you won't slip. Place a stool or a pillow on the floor beneath you so you can slide down the wall when you're finished and sit on it if you need to. Cross your arms over your chest or hold your elbows. Tighten your abdominals.

Slowly lower your body to a count of 8, bending your knees and rolling the ball along your back. Bring your thighs parallel to the floor. Pause in this position for a moment, squeezing your behind to intensify the hold. Keep your abdominals tight. Then s-l-o-w-l-y push back up the wall to a count of 8.

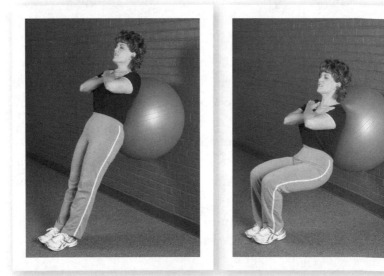

Breathe deeply and exhale as you push back up. Don't straighten your legs completely at the top. Repeat for approximately 2 minutes or until muscle failure.

When you're ready for more of a challenge, add 3 to 5 pound hand weights.

Scriptural affirmation to meditate on: God made me alive with Christ (by grace I have been saved), and raised me up, and made me sit in the heavenly places in Christ Jesus! (Ephesians 2:5-6).

4. *Push-ups.* Push-ups work not only the chest muscles and arms but also the back, abdomen, and legs. Start with a beginner's push-up (with your knees on the floor). Place a folded towel under your knees for added comfort. Position your hands directly under your shoulders. Keep your back straight and your abdomen tight. Tuck in your chin slightly to avoid craning or injuring your neck.

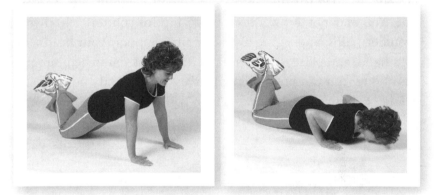

Start the push-up with your arms straight (but not locked), inhale, and slowly lower your body to the floor to a count of 8. Pause briefly when your chest touches the floor, then exhale as you push back up to the very slow count of 8. Don't rest at the bottom of the motion; immediately begin to push back up to the starting position. Don't lock your elbows when you reach the top. Breathe gently, and don't hold your breath or contort your face. When you're confident you're performing the push-up correctly, say the scripture aloud or meditate on it.

If the beginner's push-up becomes too easy, advance to the classic push-up with your legs straight behind you. If you're not strong enough yet to do either, start in the beginner's position and slowly lower yourself to the floor. Then instead of pushing back up to the starting position, get back there in a way that's easiest for you. Once you're back in position, slowly lower yourself to the floor again. In time you'll develop more upper-body strength and be able to push back up while on your knees.

If you prefer, you can stand and push off slowly from a wall.

Continue with the proper form for 2 minutes or until muscle failure.

Scripture to meditate on: "I press toward the goal for the prize of the upward call of God in Christ Jesus" (Philippians 3:14).

5. *Weighted leg lifts.* Put on your ankle weights, unless the weight of your own leg is sufficient to get a good workout. Lie on your side. You may put a towel under your hip for comfort. Keep your shoulders, hips, and legs in a straight line. Support your head with your hand, and place the other hand in front of you to help support your body. You can put a pillow between your hand and head if it would be more comfortable. Tighten your abdominals.

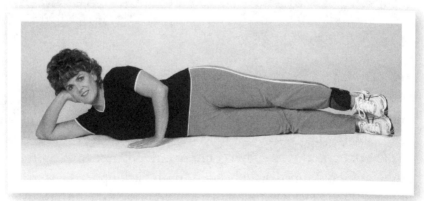

Flex your foot (toes toward you) and slowly raise your leg from the hip as high as you can. Take a full 8 counts to reach the top.

Squeeze your leg at the top of the lift before lowering slowly to a count of 8. Do not rest your leg at the bottom, but immediately begin to raise it again. Add the scripture when you're confident of your form during the exercise.

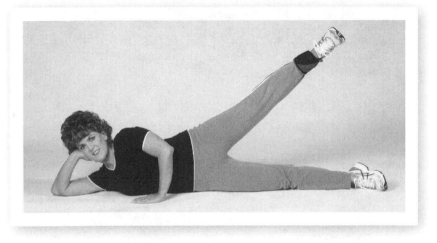

Breathe gently and evenly throughout the exercise. Continue for 2 minutes, or until muscle failure. Repeat on the other side.

Scriptural affirmation to meditate on: I am strong and of good courage. I am not afraid or dismayed, for the Lord my God is with me wherever I go (Joshua 1:9).

6. *Back extension/leg lifts.* Lie facedown on a towel or an exercise mat. Straighten your arms and place them under your upper thighs with your palms up. Keep your abdominals tight to protect your lower back.

Inhale. Exhale as you slowly lift your shoulders and legs to a count of 8. When you reach the top of the lift, squeeze your leg muscles and buttocks for a few seconds and then slowly lower your legs and shoulders back to the floor to a count of 8.

Don't rest at the bottom of the motion. Slowly begin to lift your shoulders and legs again. Continue the exercise for 2 minutes or until muscle failure. Add the scripture when you're confident you're doing the exercise correctly.

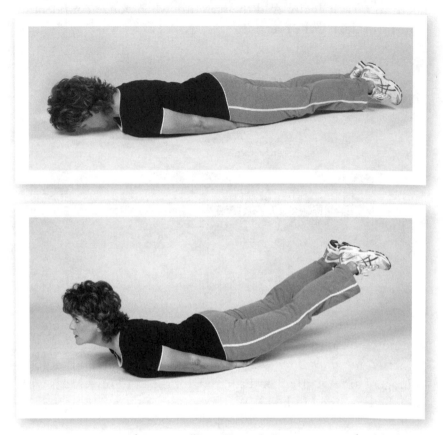

Scripture to meditate on: "But You, O Lᴏʀᴅ, are a shield about me, my glory, and the lifter of my head" (Psalm 3:3 ᴇꜱᴠ).

7. *Abdominal crunches.* Lie on your back with your knees bent and your feet flat on the floor. Place your fingers behind your head and your thumbs by your temples or jaw. You'll lift up using only your abdominal muscles. Do *not* jerk your neck up. Keep your head cradled in your hands, elbows out to the sides. Push your lower back into the floor and look up at the ceiling as you slowly lift your chest and shoulders off the floor to a count of 8. Keep your head in the

same position, cradled in your hands, while looking straight up at the ceiling, not forward. Breathe gently and evenly throughout the exercise. Don't hold your breath. Keep your face and neck relaxed.

When you reach the top of the lift, squeeze your abdominal muscles for a moment and then slowly lower back to the floor to a count of 8.

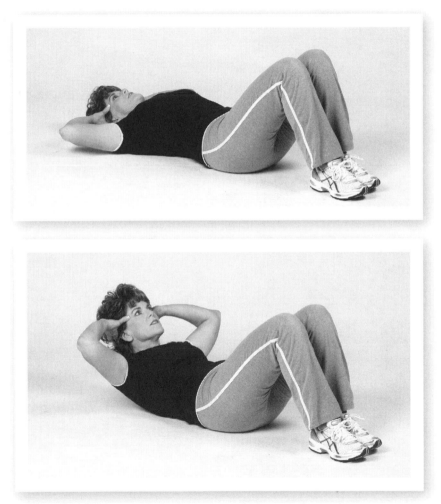

Add the scripture when you're comfortable with the exercise and are sure you're maintaining the proper form.

Scriptural affirmation to meditate on: I lay aside every weight and the sin which so easily ensnares me, and I run with endurance the race that is set before me, looking unto Jesus, the author and finisher of my faith (Hebrews 12:1-2).

MAKING IT PERSONAL

1. According to a study in the *American Journal of Clinical Nutrition,* "Although _____ minutes of daily moderate-intensity physical activity may result in significant improvements in health, it appears that progressing to at least _____ minutes of physical activity may be necessary for enhancing long-term weight loss outcomes."

2. Two ways we may strengthen the fruit of the Spirit in our lives is by _____ to the Holy Spirit and His fruit and by _____ seeds of patience, faithfulness, self-control (or love, joy, peace, kindness, goodness, gentleness).

3. One way I can develop the fruit of _____ in my life is to

_____

_____ when I am tempted to do otherwise.

4. This week I will do these Slow-Cadence exercises:_____

_____

_____

PRAISEMOVES®— THE CHRISTIAN ALTERNATIVE TO YOGA

*You were bought with a price;
therefore glorify God in your body and
in your spirit, which are God's.*

1 CORINTHIANS 6:20

Why do we need a Christian alternative to yoga? Isn't yoga just a series of flexibility exercises? Yes, but unfortunately yoga does far more than stretch the body. In *Webster's New World Dictionary,* "yoga" (coming from an east Indian Sanskrit word that means "union with god" or "to yoke") is described as "a mystic and ascetic Hindu discipline for achieving union with the supreme spirit through meditation, prescribed postures, controlled breathing, etc." Doesn't this sound like an attempt to achieve salvation by works instead of grace?

In our culture the more pervasive and visible something becomes, the more accepted it is. In the past 50 years yoga has gone from being a relatively unknown Hindu practice to part of our mainstream culture. Those who think yoga is little more than a series of stress-relieving stretching exercises may be surprised to learn about the true foundation of the multibillion-dollar yoga craze in North America.

As a child growing up on Long Island, I became involved with yoga at the age of 7 when my mother and I began watching a daily yoga exercise program on television. For the next 22 years I was heavily involved with yoga, metaphysics, and the New Age move-ment...until I came to the end of myself and surrendered my life to Jesus Christ in 1987.

I call yoga the missionary arm of Hinduism and the New Age movement. From experience I can say that yoga is a dangerous practice for Christians and leads seekers *away* from God rather than to Him. You may say, "Well, I'm not doing any of the chanting or meditation stuff. I'm just doing the exercises." Even so, it's impossible to separate yoga the technique from yoga the religion.

Yoga Postures: Offerings to 330 Million Gods

You may have heard proponents of yoga say, "It's only exercise" or "Yoga is *science,* not religion." But what do Hindus and true Yogis (adherents of Yogic philosophy) say? In an article in *Time Magazine,* "Stretching for Jesus,"[1] Subhas Tiwari, a professor of yoga philosophy and meditation at the Hindu University of America in Orlando, Florida, was quoted as saying, "Yoga is Hinduism." In the same article, I am quoted as saying that "Christian yoga is an oxymoron" (a contradiction in terms, such as a Christian Buddhist).

Yoga postures are actually offerings to 330 million Hindu gods. Can you see the subtle satanic twist of Romans 12:1, *"Present your bodies* a living sacrifice"? One of our PraiseMoves instructors spent three months on a missionary trip to India several years ago. She said her group often saw people performing yoga postures in front of statues of the gods in the streets. Some brought offerings of flowers, some fruit, and some even presented *themselves* as offerings.

Acts 15:29 tells us to "abstain from *things* offered to idols."

In an article titled "Bible, Yoga Strike a Pose," Sannyasin Aru-mugaswami, managing editor of *Hinduism Today,* said that Hinduism is the soul of yoga, "based as it is on Hindu Scripture and developed by Hindu sages. Yoga opens up new and more refined states of mind, and to understand them one needs to believe in and understand the Hindu way of looking at God...A Christian trying to adapt these practices will likely disrupt their own Christian beliefs."[2]

Sadly, many well-intentioned believers teach "Christian yoga" classes, and there are even books and DVDs by Christians on the subject. One book/DVD claims that Christian yoga offers a "Christ-centered approach to physical and *spiritual* health" (emphasis added).[3] Even though proponents of Christian yoga might say their Christ-centered approach eliminates any concerns about the potential influences of Hindu philosophy, I disagree. An inherently Hindu-centered approach cannot also be Christ-centered. Christian yoga is an example of *syncretism,* the blending of conflicting beliefs, religions, and philosophies.

Perhaps you or someone you love studies or teaches yoga (or "Christian" yoga). You may believe it's completely compatible with your Christian faith and feel your relationship with the Lord is unshakable. I ask you to consider for a moment the young Christians and nonbelievers in your life who are influenced by your actions. Might they be drawn into yoga and the New Age movement (like my mother and I were) because they've been led to believe that it's "only exercise"?

PraiseMoves®: A Christ-Centered Alternative

I'm so grateful the Lord gave me the idea for PraiseMoves—The Christian *Alternative* to Yoga. This program is designed to help you build strength and flexibility in your body, renew your mind by meditating on the Word of God, and nourish your spirit as you praise the Lord. Using this approach you can experience all the benefits of stretching and flexibility exercises with the added bonus of meditating on God's Word.

I cry tears of joy just about every time people send me testimonies of how the Lord has used PraiseMoves to touch them physically and spiritually. I believe this program touches them spiritually as well as physically because the foundation of PraiseMoves is the Word of God, not the postures. The postures are merely witty inventions designed to draw people into a deeper relationship with the Lord through His Word. Since so many doctors are recommending yoga, it's exciting to offer a Christ-centered alternative that delivers the same or better results than yoga! The physical benefits of PraiseMoves are: improved flexibility; weight loss; reduced stress; improved circulation, coordination, and agility; improved bone and tissue health; and better healing of injuries. By reducing stress and promoting a healthy lifestyle and a positive attitude, PraiseMoves can also help soften the transition through the menopausal years.

BUSY WOMAN'S QUICK TIP
CBA—CORRECT BODY ALIGNMENT

Posture is important. Many of our daily activities cause our bodies to slump forward, putting strain on our neck and shoulders. Sitting at the computer, caring for children, washing dishes, vacuuming, even pushing a shopping cart has us leaning forward, our shoulders hunched, our lungs compressed, and our tummies "pooched" out. Correct body alignment (CBA) helps keep you straight and tall whether you're standing or sitting. You'll get more out of your workouts, too. (The QuickFits shoulder rolls exercise presented in chapter 6 also provides this information.)

Follow these steps to ensure that your body is correctly aligned:

- Stand with your feet several inches apart and place your weight on the outsides of your feet. (This helps take pressure off the knees.) Keep your knees slightly bent.

- If you're seated, make sure your feet are flat on the floor.

- Gently tighten your abdominal muscles and tuck your pelvis under (instead of sticking out your behind and compressing the lower back).

- Slowly roll your shoulders forward and then roll them

back, rotating your arms so that your palms are facing out (away from your body) and your thumbs are pointing behind you. Do this several times so you can feel the difference between gently rolling your shoulders back and throwing your shoulders straight back and sticking your chest out, which you don't want to do. Breathe gently and evenly.

- Again, roll your shoulders forward, then back, with your palms facing out. This time *keep your shoulders in the same rolled-back position* as you slowly rotate your arms so that your palms are facing your body again. Relax your arms, neck, and shoulders, but make sure you keep your shoulders rolled back.

- Lift up through the crown of your head so that your chin is parallel with the floor. See if you can make yourself an inch taller. Keep your shoulders in the same rolled-back position.

That's perfect posture! Now when you feel your shoulders slump forward again, simply roll them back and let your arms come to your sides. Breathe gently and deeply, making sure you keep your abdominal muscles engaged (not "pooched out").

PraiseMoves® Postures

PraiseMoves postures are gentle stretches you can do at home to make the most out of 20 minutes and transform your workout into worship.

Wear loose, comfortable clothing for your workout and keep a glass of pure drinking water handy to stay well hydrated. After eating, wait one or two hours before starting your PraiseMoves workout. You'll want to work out in a warm space free of distractions. Proceed at a relaxed pace. Let this be your special time with the Lord and His Word. Be gentle with yourself while doing PraiseMoves.

Remember that you're coaxing your body to become more flexible. Never force a stretch.

Breathe smoothly and deeply into the lower and upper lungs as you perform the PraiseMoves postures. Inhale as you go into a posture and exhale as you come out of it. Avoid holding your breath. (See chapter 7 if you need a refresher on diaphragmatic breathing.) If you become light-headed, sit or lie down and rest.

One way to keep track of your breathing, as well as how long you're holding a stretch, is to inhale for 5 seconds and then exhale for 5 seconds. If you hold each posture for 3 to 5 complete breaths, you'll be holding each posture for 30 to 50 seconds. Don't hold a stretch for more than 50 to 60 seconds.

Accompanying each posture is a scripture you can either speak aloud or meditate on silently.

These 12 basic PraiseMoves postures and more are presented on the *PraiseMoves* DVD (see Resources for more information).

1. *Mount Zion.* Stand with your feet a few inches apart. Bend your knees slightly. Rest your weight on the outsides of your feet. Tuck your pelvis under and tighten your abdominal muscles. Keep your shoulders rotated back and reach down with your fingers. Lift up through the crown of your head as if you're trying to add another inch to your height.

Scripture to meditate on: "Those who trust in the Lord are like Mount Zion, which cannot be moved, but abides forever" (Psalm 125:1).

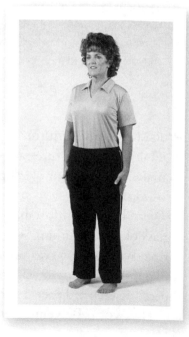

2. *The Reed.* Sweep your hands forward, clasping your thumbs together and reaching upward. Keep your pelvis tucked under to protect your lower back. Bring your upper arms alongside your ears. Raise your head and look up at the ceiling.

Scripture to meditate on: "A bruised reed He will not break, and smoking flax He will not quench" (Isaiah 42:3).

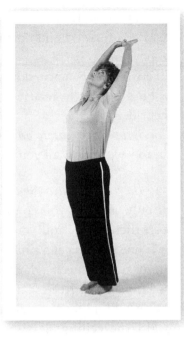

3. *The Angel.* Bring one leg behind you, heel to the floor. Bend the knee of the leg in front so your knee aligns with your ankle. Keep your abdominals tight. Breathe gently. Raise your arms overhead and slowly stretch from your hips and waist all the way up through

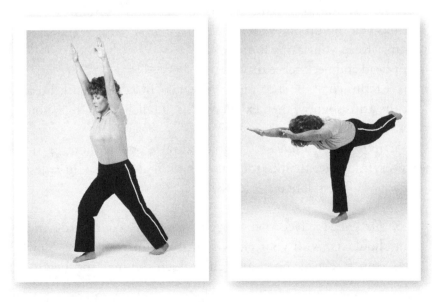

your fingertips. If you can, bring your upper arms alongside your ears. Look forward and down slightly, keeping your head in a neutral position.

To work on balance, slowly lift your back leg behind you bit by bit. Find a point to focus on as you build balance. Repeat on the other side.

Scripture to meditate on: "He shall give His angels charge over you, to keep you in all your ways" (Psalm 91:11).

4. *The Tallit (Prayer Shawl).* When doing this stretch, go slowly and only as far as you comfortably can. Bring your chin to your chest, then slowly roll your body down one vertebra at a time. Keep your head and neck relaxed and your arms loose. Keep your knees slightly bent, tailbone reaching up toward the ceiling. If you want more of a stretch, you can fold your arms over your chest.

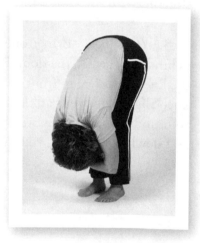

Come out of The Tallit posture very slowly, pulling in your abdomen as you roll up one vertebra at a time. Keep your arms limp and your head and neck relaxed. When you've returned to the starting posture, take in a deep, gentle breath, lift the arms slightly, then exhale with a "Hallelujah." That should feel *very* good!

Scripture to meditate on: "Rejoice always, pray without ceasing, in everything give thanks; for this is the will of God in Christ Jesus for you" (1 Thessalonians 5:16-18).

5. *The Vine.* Lie facedown on your mat. Place your hands under your shoulders, with your elbows tucked into your sides. Slowly glide your forehead, nose, and chin along the mat and begin to

raise your head, look-
ing up toward the ceiling.
Keep your elbows bent
and pressed into your sides.
Keep your hipbones on the
floor. Look up at the ceiling, pressing your chest
forward. Breathe deeply.

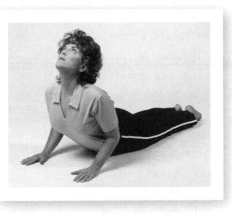

Scripture to meditate on:
"[Jesus said,] I am the vine,
you are the branches. He
who abides in Me, and I in him, bears much fruit; for without Me
you can do nothing" (John 15:5).

6. *The Little Child.* Begin facedown on your abdomen with
your legs together. Push
your body up into a sitting
posture on your haunches,
keeping your knees
together and underneath
you. Slowly bend forward,
lowering your body until
your forehead is resting on
the floor. Move your arms
to your sides or overhead
and rest them on the floor.

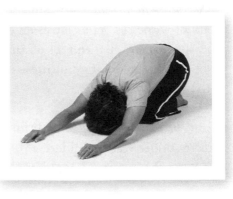

Relax your face and neck. To modify this posture, you can sit on a
pillow or spread your knees apart if that's more comfortable.

Scripture to meditate on: "[Jesus said,] Assuredly, I say to you,
whoever does not receive the kingdom of God as a little child will
by no means enter it" (Mark 10:15).

7. *The Runner.* Begin on your hands and knees with your arms
directly under your shoulders. Bring one leg forward until your

foot is positioned between your hands. Extend the other leg behind you in a runner's stretch. Bring your hips down. If you prefer, you can place your back knee on the floor. Keep your weight on your fingertips, palms, or fists. Your head and neck should remain in a neutral position. Breathe gently and evenly.

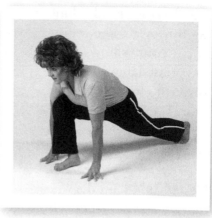

Slowly straighten both legs while keeping your fingers in contact with the floor. Bring your forehead to your front knee. You'll feel the stretch primarily in the hamstring muscles of your front leg. Repeat on the other side.

Scripture to meditate on: "Since we are surrounded by so great a cloud of witnesses, let us lay aside every weight, and the sin which so easily ensnares us, and let us run with endurance the race that is set before us, looking unto Jesus, the author and finisher of our faith" (Hebrews 12:1-2).

8. *The Flapping Tent.* On all fours, with your hands positioned directly under your shoulders, inhale, letting your tailbone tilt up and your spine curve downward. Look up at the ceiling. Exhale,

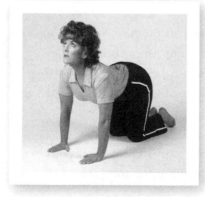
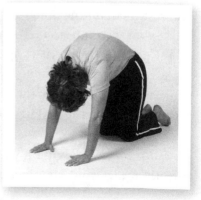

reversing the spinal bend, tilting your tailbone downward and pulling your chest and your abdomen in. Like the wind coming in and out of a tent, flow from one posture to the other.

Scripture to meditate on: "The Spirit of God has made me, and the breath of the Almighty gives me life" (Job 33:4).

9. *The Tent.* Get on your hands and knees, with toes contacting the floor underneath you (not pointing), legs hip-width apart, and arms shoulder-width apart about a foot in front of you. Spread your fingers wide apart, with your middle fingers parallel to each other, pointing straight ahead. Rotate the inside of your elbows forward. With your arms

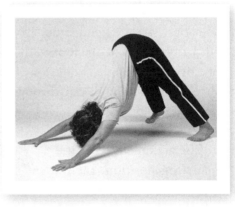

straight (but not locked), slowly begin to raise your hips up and back, reaching your tailbone toward the ceiling and straightening your legs. Keep your head in a neutral position. Press your heels toward the floor for an added calf stretch. You can bend your knees slightly to help straighten your back. Remember to breathe gently throughout the exercise.

Bend your knees to come out of The Tent and come down to The Little Child posture.

Scripture to meditate on: "Enlarge the place of your tent, and let them stretch out the curtains of your dwellings; do not spare; lengthen your cords, and strengthen your stakes" (Isaiah 54:2).

10. *The Altar.* Begin on all fours with your hands directly under your shoulders, your fingers spread apart. Straighten one leg behind you, then the other, bringing your body into a straight line and keeping your toes in contact with the floor. Breathe gently and

evenly. Keep your abdominals tight, your hips down, and your head in a neutral position.

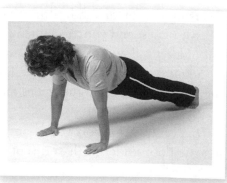

Scripture to meditate on: "I beseech you therefore, brethren, by the mercies of God, that you present your bodies a living sacrifice, holy, acceptable to God, which is your reasonable service" (Romans 12:1).

11. *The Prayer Warrior.* Begin in a standing position with legs wide apart, arms extended out to your sides, palms down. Inhale and turn the toes of one foot to the side, then exhale, bending that knee over your ankle. Look toward the bent knee, then out over your fingertips. Reach out through your fingertips, keeping your hips and shoulders facing forward. Breathe deeply into the abdomen. Return to starting position, then repeat on the other side.

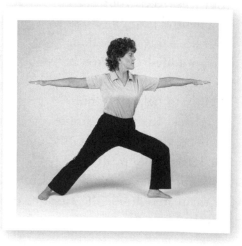

Scripture to meditate on: "Confess your trespasses to one another, and pray for one another, that you may be healed. The effective, fervent prayer of a righteous man avails much" (James 5:16).

12. *The Tree.* Place the instep of one foot over the top of the other. Bend your supporting knee slightly. Keep your abdominals tight and your pelvis tucked under. Inhale slowly, then exhale, lifting your

arms overhead like the branches of a tree, ending with your palms upward or facing one another. Repeat on the other side.

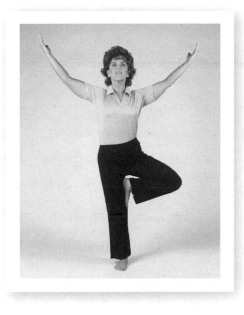

To build balance, place one foot on the inside of your calf or thigh (not the knee). Focus your eyes on one spot in front of you to keep your balance, and then reach your arms up. Keep your bent knee pressed back to ensure that your thigh and hip stay open. Repeat on the other side.

Scripture to meditate on: "[A righteous man] shall be like a tree planted by the rivers of water, that brings forth its fruit in its season, whose leaf also shall not wither; and whatever he does shall prosper" (Psalm 1:3).

BUSY WOMAN'S QUICK TIP
SPEEDY 20-MINUTE WORKOUTS

How many ways can you combine spiritual and physical fitness in a busy schedule? Plenty!

- Enjoy a walk with your family or a friend and discuss a scripture or Bible story.
- Work out to the *PraiseMoves* DVD (see Resources).

- Combine the Gimme Ten Workout (10-minute exercises with light weights and the Word) with a brisk cardio walk or a 10-minute PraiseMoves session (see Resources).

- Experience a Slow-Cadence Exercise (SCE) workout (see chapter 8).

- Read a devotional while walking on the treadmill.

- Bounce on a rebounder (a mini-trampoline) or jog in place while listening to praise music, meditating on Scripture, or speaking scriptural affirmations aloud.

- Take a brisk 20-minute walk outdoors or work out on a treadmill, stationary bike, or rowing machine while you pray and meditate on Scripture. Another suggestion is to follow the ten steps of the Lord's Prayer presented in my book *BASIC Steps to Godly Fitness* under "A Daily Walk with the Lord's Prayer."

- Take a prayer walk. One biblical example of prayer walking is Isaac, who "went out to meditate in the field."[4] Eighteenth-century English evangelist George Müller also wrote, "I find it very beneficial to my health to walk thus for meditation before breakfast, and... generally take out a New Testament...and I find that I can profitably spend my time in the open air."[5] Pray for family, friends, and neighbors as you walk. Meditate on God's Word or bring along an index card with Bible verses written on it. Other prayer-walking options include taking a brisk prayer walk as part of your daily lunch hour, wearing a pedometer and purposing to walk 10,000 steps a day, and setting a goal to walk or ride a bike for a worthy charity you're also committed to praying for.

MAKING IT PERSONAL

1. In the words of many Christians and Hindus, including Hindu yoga professor Subhas Tiwari, quoted in *Time* magazine, "Yoga is _____."

2. Yoga postures are actually _____ to 330 million Hindu gods.

3. Acts 15:29 tells us to "abstain from _____ offered to idols."

4. I especially like the scripture that accompanies the _____ posture. It reads, "_____ _____," from _____.

21 DAYS TO TOTAL FITNESS WITH THE VIRTUOUS ("MIGHTY") WOMAN

Every part of Scripture is God-breathed and useful one way or another— showing us truth, exposing our rebellion, correcting our mistakes, training us to live God's way.

2 TIMOTHY 3:16 MSG

When we think of a busy woman in Scripture, many of us agree the "Virtuous Woman" of Proverbs 31 definitely qualifies. We can learn a lot from her, but several women have told me she makes them feel guilty, inadequate, and even angry. One woman commented, "She makes the rest of us look bad. How can I possibly measure up?" Well, that's certainly not the Lord's intention!

As I've studied Scripture, I've found that learning the definitions of certain words in their original languages gives me deeper and more personal insights into passages such as Proverbs 31. As this chapter's opening verse from 2 Timothy illustrates, God's Word is a mirror of sorts, "showing us truth, exposing our rebellion, correcting our mistakes, training us to live God's way."

Let's focus on the final 22 verses of Proverbs 31. In 21 daily devotional studies, we'll explore various aspects of the biblical busy woman in this passage and discover why the original Hebrew calls her *eshet chayil,* "mighty or powerful woman." Although many translations call her "a virtuous *wife*," in the original Hebrew the word *eshet* means "woman." As such, she serves as an example not only for married women but also for single women, single moms, widows, and any other woman who doesn't fit into these categories. We'll also learn what this virtuous woman can teach us about how "to live God's way." I've chosen to use the Amplified version of the Bible for our discussion of Proverbs 31 because it references the original Hebrew to expand our understanding.

Proverbs 31:10-31 is an acrostic passage. An *acrostic* is a poem or psalm in which each verse or group of verses starts with or forms a letter of the alphabet, a word, or a name. For example, in Psalm 119, the Bible's longest psalm, every eight verses begin with a different letter of the Hebrew alphabet, from *alef* through *tav* (we would say A to Z). Your Bible may even show these Hebrew letters at the start of each series of eight verses. Likewise, the last 22 verses of Proverbs 31 about the virtuous woman follow the same progression—each verse beginning with a different letter of the Hebrew alphabet in sequential order—*alef* through *tav*.

Some Bible experts say that acrostics were used to help in the memorization of these portions of Scripture. Others believe we can gain new insights into these acrostic passages when we study the pictures these Hebrew letters paint for us.

I'm constantly amazed by how multifaceted the Lord is! He never ceases to astonish me with revelations of His goodness and grace. As we study this busy woman of Proverbs 31, I pray He will continue to amaze us.

PraiseMoves Alphabetics and Hebrew Word Pictures

Along with the daily devotionals in this chapter, I've included 21 mini-workouts to round out your Total Fitness journey. These workouts will incorporate a wonderful series of 22 postures called PraiseMoves Alphabetics, which mirror the Hebrew alphabet, as well as a PraiseMoves posture, a Slow-Cadence Exercise, or a QuickFits Workout. (There are approximately 60 basic PraiseMoves postures with corresponding scriptures, and more are being created all the time. We have some *very* gifted certified PraiseMoves instructors!)

BUSY WOMAN'S QUICK TIP
DEVOTIONS IN MOTION

Each daily devotion and mini-workout is designed to be completed in 20 minutes or less; however, for added benefit, you may want to add the following:

- Read a chapter from the New Testament every day.

- Praise and worship the Lord; ask for His guidance and listen.

- Pray for your nation's leaders, the body of Christ around the world, your church family, and your pastor.

- Repeat the exercises several times.

- Take a brisk walk when you have a little extra time.

At one time Hebrew was an ideogrammatic language in which pictures represented words. Biblical Hebrew is still full of many powerful word pictures that clearly illustrate the truths of the Bible. Although we have to be careful in applying today's views to ancient words, we can get some fascinating insights. For example, in Hebrew the word for "father" is *abba* (actually a closer translation would be "dad" or "daddy," since *ab* or *av* represents "father"). This word is actually a combination of the first and second letters of the Hebrew alphabet, *alef* and *bet*. The word *alef* means "ox," "strength," or "first," and the word *bet* means "house," "home," or "family" (as in *Bet*hlehem, which means "the *House* of Bread"). So *abba* ("father") can mean "the strength of the home" or "the strength of the family."

Can you see how the study of God's Word becomes even more fascinating when we explore it in light of the original languages?[1] We'll look at a few more as we go along.

Let's begin our three-week Total Fitness journey with the virtuous woman!

> When exercising it's important to not overdo. If an exercise causes pain (not just mild discomfort), don't continue to do it. If you have physical problems, be careful to modify or avoid the exercises that might aggravate your condition.

21 DAYS TO TOTAL FITNESS

Day 1

Scripture for today. "A capable, intelligent, and virtuous woman—who is he who can find her? She is far more precious than jewels and her value is far above rubies or pearls" (Proverbs 31:10 AMP).

Insights into the Word. In Hebrew the phrase translated "virtuous woman" (or "virtuous wife" in some versions) was *eshet chayil,* which means "a powerful or mighty woman." As it's used in the Old Testament, *chayil* means "able," "power," "wealth," and "strength."

If you're like me, you often don't feel very powerful or mighty (and sometimes not very capable or intelligent either). The good news is that "God has chosen the weak things of the world to put to shame the things which are mighty,"[2] and because Christ's strength is made perfect in our weakness, we can say with the apostle Paul, "When I am weak, then I am strong."[3]

Lord, my prayer today is… "Father God, my 'natural self' often feels small and insignificant. Without You I can do nothing, but with You all things are possible. I choose not to be strong in my own might but to lean on You completely today. By turning to You and choosing to follow as You lead me by Your Word and by the inward guidance of Your Holy Spirit, I will have the strength to meet any challenge that comes my way.

"Who is the one who can find a virtuous woman? Lord, I pray it's You. I pray that You will find a virtuous woman in me today. I place myself in Your Potter's hands and ask You to mold me into the person You have called me to be so I will bring You glory and honor in Jesus' name. Amen."

ℵ Mini-Workout
PraiseMoves Alphabetics: Alef—The Ox
("Strength, Leader, First")

On all fours, slowly raise your right leg toward the ceiling with your knee bent. Hold this pos-

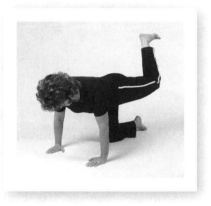

ture for a moment, then lower your leg. Keep your abdominals tight and your back straight. Your head should remain in neutral position. Breathe gently and evenly. Repeat several times, then switch to the left leg as you meditate on the scripture.

Meditate on today's scripture (Proverbs 31:10).

Slow-Cadence Exercise™: Push-Ups

Start in a push-up position with your hands directly under your shoulders, your arms straight (but not locked), and your legs extended. (If a classic push-up is too difficult for you right now, start on your knees until you build up enough upper-body strength.) Keep your back straight and your abdomen tight. Tuck in your chin slightly to avoid craning or injuring your neck. Inhale as you slowly lower your body to the floor to a count of 8.

Pause briefly when your chest touches the floor, then exhale as you push back up at a very slow count of 8. Don't rest at the bottom of the motion; immediately begin to push back up to the starting position. Don't lock your elbows when you reach the top. Breathe gently and don't hold your breath or contort your face. Repeat the scripture when you're confident you're performing the push-up correctly.

Continue with the proper form for 2 minutes or until muscle failure.

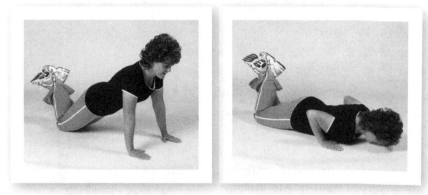

Scripture to meditate on: "I press toward the goal for the prize of the upward call of God in Christ Jesus" (Philippians 3:14).

Day 2

Scripture for today. "The heart of her husband trusts in her confidently and relies on and believes in her securely, so that he has no lack of [honest] gain or need of [dishonest] spoil" (Proverbs 31:11 AMP, brackets in original).

Insights into the Word. I prefer the New King James wording for this verse: "The heart of her husband *safely trusts* her." When someone safely trusts in you, it's because you've proven yourself to be faithful and reliable. This trust is based on relationship and experience gained over time. There's power in that relationship, which is why the enemy does all he can to put enmity and strife between a wife and her husband.

There's tremendous power available to a couple who prays.

When a husband and wife agree in prayer, the Lord is in their midst ("Where two or three are gathered together in My name, I am there in the midst of them").[4] Where there's strife and lack of forgiveness, prayers can be hindered,[5] as they can be if a husband doesn't honor his wife.[6]

When a husband and wife are allies, "he will have no lack of gain." Indeed, their relationship will flourish and prosper, and the wife will have no lack of gain either.

Lord, my prayer today is... "Heavenly Father, I pray that I'll be a person worthy of the trust of those who love me—my husband, children, family, and friends. I also choose to be a trustworthy person in other areas of my everyday life, whether it's working on the job, shopping at a store, driving the car, surfing the Internet, or paying bills. Whatever I'm called to do, give me the grace to do it with excellence and in a trustworthy manner. I choose to operate in a way worthy of the trust You have obviously placed in me. Help me treat the people and things in my life responsibly as gifts from You. Thank You, Lord, for trusting in me. I'm grateful for that trust and purpose to walk worthy of it today. I pray in Jesus' name. Amen."

ℶ Mini-Workout
PraiseMoves Alphabetics: Bet—The Home
("Household, in, into, Family")

Sit up straight on the floor, your legs together and out in front of you and your feet flexed (toes pointing toward the ceiling). Stretch your arms out straight in front of you with your palms flexed. Lean forward slightly over your legs, keeping your abdominals tight. Breathe deeply.

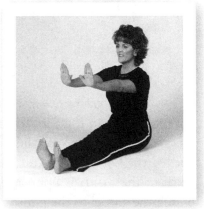

Meditate on today's scripture (Proverbs 31:11).

PraiseMoves Posture: The Scroll

Sit up straight on the floor with your legs out in front of you. Place your hands on the top of your thighs, then bend forward over your legs, keeping your back straight and your abdominals tight. Look up at the ceiling until you've come as far as you comfortably can. Then let your head and neck relax and let your torso go limp over your legs. Breathe gently and deeply.

With each exhalation, see if you can go just one millimeter deeper into the stretch.

Slowly round your body up to the starting position, then repeat the stretch with one leg out in front of you and the opposite leg bent, with the foot pressed into your thigh. Hold for a few breaths, then switch legs and repeat. Finally, with both legs comfortably apart (in a V), gently walk your hands along the floor in front of you. Relax. Put your weight on your hands as you slowly round back up at starting position.

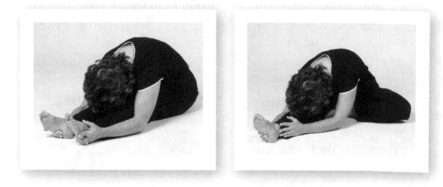

Scripture to meditate on: "As His custom was, [Jesus] went into the synagogue on the Sabbath day, and stood up to read. And He was handed the book of the prophet Isaiah. And when He had opened the book, He found the place where it was written: 'The Spirit of the LORD is upon Me, because He has anointed Me to preach the gospel to the poor'" (Luke 4:16-18).

Day 3

Scripture for today. "She comforts, encourages, and does him only good as long as there is life within her" (Proverbs 31:12 AMP).

Insights into the Word. You've probably heard that Eve was taken from Adam's side for a reason: not from his head to be above him, nor from his feet to be beneath him, but from his side to be equal to him. Only an equal—an ally, a partner, and an intimate friend—can truly comfort and encourage us. The Holy Spirit is called our Comforter, the *parakletos,* which means "advocate," "intercessor," or "one called to come alongside." Although we can never come close to the perfection of the Holy Spirit, we can see the great love and power in a woman's God-given ability to comfort, encourage, and do good.

When I look at the word "encourage," I see the word "courage," from the French word for "heart." When we encourage and give people hope, we're adding courage and strength to their hearts. We all know how much better we feel when we know someone believes in us, especially when we're feeling a little shaky. Who can you encourage today? Ask the Lord. Is there a scripture you can share with that person? Ask the Lord to give you the words to say that will be a blessing.

Lord, my prayer today is… "Heavenly Father, help me be a comfort and encourager to my family and those I meet today. Comfort them through me. Encourage them and add goodness to them through me. As a channel for Your blessing, I know it's 'not by might nor by power, but by [Your] Spirit!'[7] Amen."

⫶ Mini-Workout
PraiseMoves Alphabetics: Gimmel—The Camel ("To Lift Up")

Starting from a kneeling position, place your right foot on the floor in front of you, knee bent. Keep your knee in line with your ankle. Bring your arms together in front of you and interlock your thumbs. Keep your abdominals tight and your pelvis tucked under. Breathe gently. Slowly bring your arms up around your ears and lean forward slightly. Bring down your arms and switch legs.

Meditate on today's scripture from Proverbs 13:12.

PraiseMoves Posture:
David's Harp

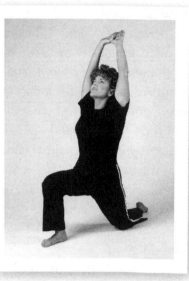

On your knees, with your body in a straight line (not sitting back on your heels), place your fists into the padded area by your hips in the back. Tighten abdominals and tuck your pelvis under. Breathe gently. Bring your elbows back as you press your body forward and look up.

To come out of the posture, slowly exhale, lifting your head to look forward first, chin to chest, and then coming up. Come up straight, not to the side. Relax into the Little Child posture (see chapter 9).

Scripture to meditate on: "Awake, lute and harp! I will awaken the dawn. I will praise You, O LORD, among the peoples, and I will sing praises to You among the nations" (Psalm 108:2-3).

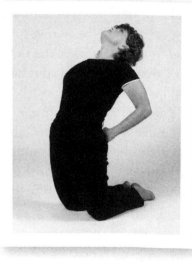

Day 4

Scripture for today. "She seeks out wool and flax and works with willing hands [to develop it]" (Proverbs 31:13 AMP, brackets in original).

Insights into the Word. Not everyone can look at a sheep and see the wool it can provide. When I look at the weedlike flax plant, the health benefits of flaxseed oil don't automatically spring to mind, let alone the lovely white-linen suit flax can become!

But God sees what we can become even when we're in our roughest, most uncultivated form. He gives us the ability to look beyond the difficult situation we're in and realize not only how far He's brought us but that He's forming strength and character in us as well. His love can also enable us to see the best in others in spite of their bad attitudes or shocking appearances.

We may not have the raw materials of wool and flax to work with, but within our grasp is "such stuff as dreams are made on."[8] Our daily experiences provide the raw materials we can fashion with willing hearts, words of encouragement, and prayer to cultivate the gardens and nurture the sheep around us.

Lord, my prayer today is… "Heavenly Father, help me see potential in every person and situation You want me to cultivate and nurture today. I trust You to give me the eyes to see and the words to say to make a difference in this world. I pray to be light in a dark place and salt to flavor someone's day with Your joy, Your peace, and Your love. Amen."

⅂ Mini-Workout

PraiseMoves Alphabetics: Dalet—
The Door ("Pathway, to Enter")

Stand with your feet together, your knees slightly bent. Bring your right arm out to the side, palm facing down. Reach your left hand behind your back and slowly work your way up until the back of your hand and fingers are as close to your right shoulder blade as you can bring them. Next, reach your right hand up and over, working your hand slowly down your back to touch your left fingertips. If needed, hold a scarf, belt, or towel in your hands to help you slowly bring your hands together. Relax your arms and switch sides, repeating the Scripture verse. Keep your abdominals tight and your pelvis tucked under. Breathe gently while performing this posture, and in time your shoulders and arms will become more flexible.

Meditate on today's scripture (Proverbs 31:13).

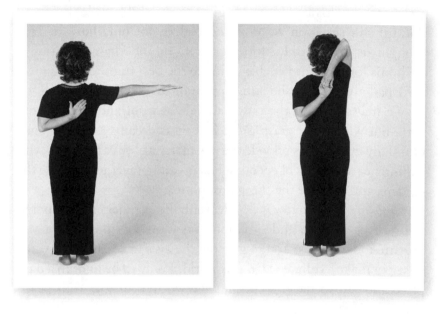

PraiseMoves Posture: The Star

Stand with your feet wide apart, toes facing outward at about 45 degrees. Keep your abdominals tight and your hips tucked under. Breathe gently and evenly. Extend your arms out to your sides and bring them up to shoulder height, palms down, reaching through the fingertips.

Variation: Tilt to one side, with one hand on your thigh and the palm of your extended hand facing forward. Pull yourself back up, reaching with your extended hand toward the ceiling. Return to starting position, then repeat on the other side.

Scripture to meditate on: "Those who are wise shall shine like the brightness of the firmament, and those who turn many to righteousness like the stars forever and ever" (Daniel 12:3).

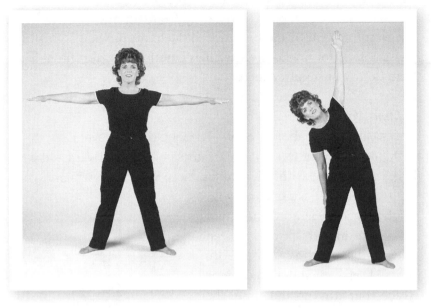

Day 5

Scripture for today. "She is like the merchant ships loaded with foodstuffs; she brings her household's food from a far [country]" (Proverbs 31:14 AMP, brackets in original).

Insights into the Word. You might be thinking, *I don't know if I like being compared to a loaded ship!* Well, of course not *physically,* but consider what a treasure of spiritual food can be for those you love.

Even though we are in this world, we're not of it. Heaven is our home, and we are here as "ambassadors for Christ."[9] The Word of God has been compared to "milk" and "solid food" ("strong meat" in the King James Version).[10] By investing time in your relationship with the Lord through studying and meditating on the "meat" of His Word, as well as praying and offering praise and worship to Him, you are filling up your spiritual storehouse. You are "a vessel for honor,"[11] laden with rich, nourishing, spiritual food you can share with your family as well as the household of believers—the household of faith!

Lord, my prayer today is… "Heavenly Father, I pray that I will be a vessel for honor. Please show me areas in my life where I'm missing the mark so I can repent (turn away from sin and turn to You), ask Your forgiveness, and be cleansed. Help me provide nourishing physical food for my family as well as emotional and spiritual food from Your vast supply. Amen."

✌ Mini-Workout
PraiseMoves Alphabetics: Hey—To Behold ("To Reveal")

Stand with your feet wide apart, toes pointing outward and your knees bent in line with your ankles. Keep your torso straight, your head in neutral position, and your pelvis tucked under. Breathe gently. Press your thighs backward to keep them as far apart as you can. Be sure to keep your abdominals tight. Reach your arms up and out to the sides, palms up. Hold this posture and breathe deeply. Return to starting position, slowly straightening your legs (but not locking your knees) and lowering your arms. Repeat.

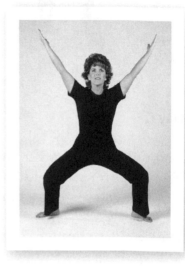

Meditate on today's scripture (Proverbs 31:14).

Slow-Cadence Exercise: Wall Slide with or without an Exercise Ball

If you don't have an exercise ball, you can still benefit from this exercise by sliding down a wall until your thighs are parallel with the floor. Hold the posture as long as you can, then slide down to sit on a stool or on pillows placed below you.

If you have an exercise ball, place it against a wall and stand with the ball against your lower back. Position your feet shoulder-width apart and move them out from the wall about 2 feet. Wear tennis shoes so you won't slip. Place a stool or a pillow on the floor beneath you so you can slide down the wall when finished and sit on it if you need to. Cross your arms over your chest or hold your elbows. Tighten your abdominals.

Slowly lower your body to a count of 8, bending your knees and rolling the ball along your back. Bring your thighs parallel to the floor. Pause in this position for a moment, squeezing your behind to intensify the hold and keeping your abdominals tight. Then s-l-o-w-l-y push back up the wall to a count of 8.

Breathe deeply and exhale as you push back up. Don't straighten your legs completely at the top. Repeat for approximately 2 minutes or until muscle failure.

When you're ready for more of a challenge, add 3- to 5-pound hand weights.

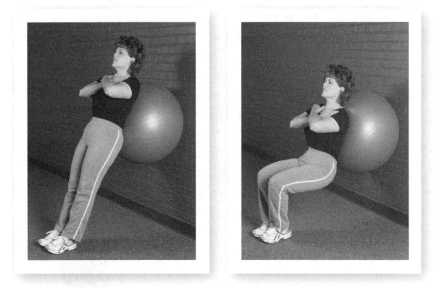

Scriptural affirmation to meditate on: God made me alive with Christ (by grace I have been saved), and raised me up, and made me sit in the heavenly places in Christ Jesus! (Ephesians 2:4-6).

Day 6

Scripture for today. "She rises while it is yet night and gets [spiritual] food for her household and assigns her maids their tasks" (Proverbs 31:15 AMP, brackets in original).

Insights into the Word. Rising while it's still night can mean before physical daylight (and I know there are many of you who do that!), yet it can also mean rising to the challenge in prayer when circumstances appear as dark as night around you. It can also refer to meeting the Lord first thing in the morning to receive guidance and insight (spiritual food) for your day.

If you're like most people, you probably don't have maids to whom you can assign daily tasks. You may, however, have friends ("maidens" or "women") with whom you can share prayer assignments ("tasks"). If you don't have a group of praying friends, ask the Lord to bring to mind one friend you can meet with on a regular basis or call for prayer and fellowship.

Lord, my prayer today is... "Heavenly Father, in the past I haven't always been faithful to seek You first. But this is a new day. I commit to turning to You before I do anything else, to say 'Good morning, Lord' first thing in my day and to look to You for guidance and direction. I trust You to provide the spiritual food my family and I need every day. Also send friends with whom I can fellowship and pray. Amen."

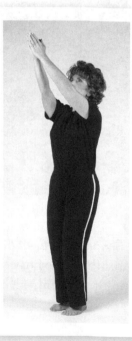

❧ *Mini-Workout*
PraiseMoves Alphabetics: Vav—
The Nail ("To Add, to Secure")

Stand with your feet together, knees slightly bent. Reach your arms forward and up, with your palms together. With your arms raised toward the ceiling, look upward past your finger-tips. Stretch up through your rib cage, holding your abdominals in and tucking your pelvis under. Breathe gently.

Meditate on today's scripture (Proverbs 31:15).

PraiseMoves Posture: The Reed

Sweep your hands forward, clasping your thumbs together and reaching upward. Tighten your abdominals and tuck your pelvis under to protect your lower back. Bring your upper arms alongside your ears. Hold this posture for a moment, looking up at the ceiling and breathing gently. Then return to starting position.

Scripture to meditate on: "A bruised reed He will not break, and smoking flax He will not quench" (Isaiah 42:3).

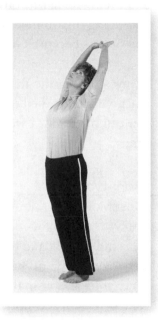

Day 7

Scripture for today. "She considers a [new] field before she buys or accepts it [expanding prudently and not courting neglect of her present duties by assuming other duties]; with her savings [of time and strength] she plants fruitful vines in her vineyard" (Proverbs 31:16 AMP, brackets in original).

Insights into the Word. It's vital to consider a new field of endeavor before taking it on. Oh boy do I know about biting off more than I can chew! How often I've taken on a new project or promised to do something before considering whether I have ample time and resources to get the task done. Just because something *needs* to be done doesn't necessarily mean we're the ones who should do it. Conversely, we shouldn't have to see rockets exploding in the air before we make a decision to move.

The busy woman is called to enter the Lord's rest and perform her work not in her own might but as unto Him, having ceased her own labors.[12] By being sensitive to the Lord's guidance, we can know when to say yes or no, when to go forward on a new project, and even whether to buy that new field (or house, stock, network-marketing distributorship). Following the Good Shepherd ensures our success because God "always leads us in triumph in Christ."[13]

Lord, my prayer today is... "Heavenly Father, thank You for always guiding me in the way I am to go. I purpose to be more sensitive and attuned to Your Holy Spirit, who leads me to do what You call me to do. I want to follow and obey Your will for my life. Amen."

↑ *Mini-Workout*
PraiseMoves Alphabetics: Zayin—
The Sword ("Cut, to Cut Off")

Stand straight and tall with your feet together, your knees slightly bent, your abdominals tight, and your pelvis tucked under. Breathe gently. Bring your arms out to your sides in line with your shoulders, your palms down. Bring your left arm across your body, barely touching your right shoulder with your left fingertips and lifting your left elbow up toward the ceiling. Turn your head to the right, looking over your fingertips. Exhale as you bring your arms down and switch to the other side.

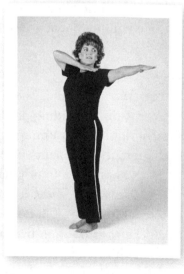

Meditate on today's scripture (Proverbs 31:16).

PraiseMoves Posture: The Rainbow

Stand with your feet shoulder-width apart, toes forward. Inhale, raising one arm with the palm up and bringing it over your head like a rainbow, ending with your palm facing down. Exhale and bend slightly to one side, feeling the stretch along your side. Keep your pelvis tucked under and your abdominals tight to protect your lower back. Breathe gently and relax.

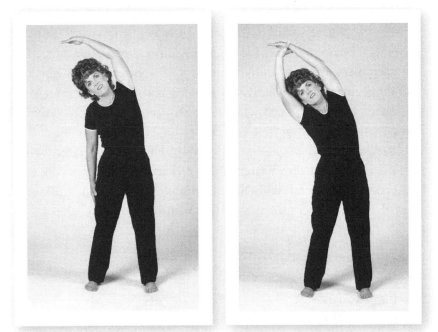

For more of a challenge, bring your opposite hand up and gently grasp the wrist of your overhead arm. Don't lean too far to the side. Lift up instead. Continue to breathe gently. Don't hold your breath. Repeat on the other side.

Scripture to meditate on: God said, "When I see the rainbow in the clouds, I will remember the eternal covenant between God and every living creature on earth" (Genesis 9:16 NLT).

Day 8

Scripture for today. "She girds herself with strength [spiritual, mental, and physical fitness for her God-given task] and makes her arms strong and firm" (Proverbs 31:17 AMP, brackets in original).

Insights into the Word. Notice that the virtuous woman girded herself with strength. She didn't expect anyone else to do her work for her. The Lord is the Source of our strength in every area of life, but we must go to Him to receive that strength.

This principle applies when we're exercising for physical strength as well. No one can work out for us. I know, I know—wouldn't it be nice if someone could? No matter what our excuses may be for not exercising, we need to realize that it's important for our health and longevity to remain active. One of my reasons for not exercising was that I hated the word "exercise"—so I changed it to "activity." Now I enjoy periods of "activity" every day. Let's get active!

Lord, my prayer today is… "Heavenly Father, I'm grateful that You are the Source of my strength. No matter what I face today or tomorrow, I know that with You all things are possible. I agree with Your Word and strengthen myself in You today. Amen."

ח *Mini-Workout*
PraiseMoves Alphabetics: Chet—
The Fence ("To Separate, Private")

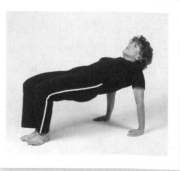

Sit on the floor and bend your knees, keeping your feet flat on the floor, your arms straight (but not locked), and your hands on the floor behind you, fingertips pointing toward your heels. Push your hips up toward the ceiling until your torso is straight across, like a table. Keep your head in neutral position. Look at the ceiling and breathe gently. Return to starting position, then repeat the posture.

Meditate on today's scripture (Proverbs 31:17).

QuickFits Workout: Triceps Extensions

Sit on the edge of your chair and lean forward slightly, keeping your back straight. Bend your elbows, pressing them into your sides, and make fists. Exhale as you lower and straighten your arms, pressing your fists back and tightening the triceps muscles on the back side of your upper arms. Hold for a count of 10 or 20, breathing gently. Relax and repeat several times. Keep your abdominals tight.

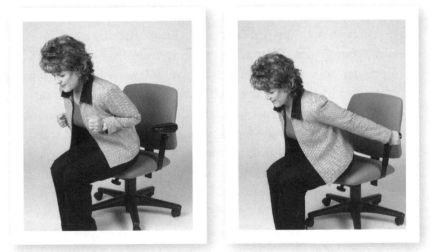

If you prefer, you can do these extensions using light weights. Instead of holding for a count of 10 to 20, you can repeat the movement back and forth with the weight for 20 to 30 repetitions.

Scriptural affirmation to meditate on: I will gird myself with strength and strengthen my arms (Proverbs 31:17).

Day 9

Scripture for today. "She tastes and sees that her gain from work [with and for God] is good; her lamp goes not out, but it burns on continually through the night [of trouble, privation, or sorrow, warning away fear, doubt, and distrust]" (Proverbs 31:18 AMP, brackets in original).

Insights into the Word. Whether you work for a company, own a business, or work at home, when your efforts are dedicated to the Lord, He is your employer. He is the Source of your supply and advancement. As you humbly trust and acknowledge Him, He will bless your labors ("Humble yourselves under the mighty hand of God, that *He may exalt you in due time,* casting all your care upon Him, *for He cares for you*").[14]

How does your work "taste" to you? Is it sweet or unsavory? Have you taken an honest look at the quality of your work recently? Have you been making gains in certain areas? Are you excelling and meeting your goals? What areas need attention?

Consider your prayer projects. Have you seen progress ("gain from work") in those areas in which you've been standing on the Word of God for a loved one's salvation, healing, deliverance, or restoration? Don't let your "lamp" go out. Keep your faith turned on and keep praising the Lord, no matter how circumstances appear.

Remember that "by faith Sarah herself also received strength... because she judged Him faithful who had promised."[15]

Lord, my prayer today is... "Heavenly Father, thank You for the work You've given me to do. This is my mission field. I trust You to give me the words to pray over my coworkers and the people You bring across my path. I will keep my switch of faith turned on, keep my 'lamp' full of the oil of the Holy Spirit, and keep it burning through the night so I may have light to help others find their way to You. Amen."

📖 Mini-Workout
PraiseMoves Alphabetics: Tet—
The Basket ("To Surround")

Sit on the floor and lean back with your arms out in front of you, your palms facing downward. Keep your abdominals tight. Breathe gently. If you can, lift your legs and balance on your coccyx (your tailbone) in a V-sit posture. Keep your back as straight as possible and your head in neutral position. Reach your arms out in front of you, palms up. For an added challenge, hold on to the outsides of your feet and balance.

Meditate on today's scripture (Proverbs 31:18).

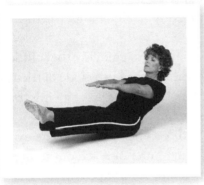 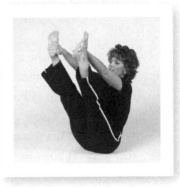

QuickFits Workout: Tummy Tuck

Sit up straight and exhale all the air out of your lungs. Now, instead of inhaling, pull in your abdominal muscles as far and as high as you can. Hold for a moment, relax, then quickly repeat. Do as many repetitions as you comfortably can without breathing. Do this exercise before eating or 1 to 2 hours after eating (for obvious reasons).

Scriptural affirmation to meditate on: My stomach shall be satisfied from the fruit of my mouth; from the produce of my lips shall I be filled (Proverbs 18:20).

Day 10

Scripture for today. "She lays her hands to the spindle, and her hands hold the distaff" (Proverbs 31:19 AMP).

Insights into the Word. This verse describes the ancient method of spinning fiber into thread in the days before the spinning wheel was invented. The *distaff* was a staff or stick on which the wool or flax was wound before spinning it on a spindle. The *spindle* was a round stick that a woman would turn or roll against her leg to twist the fibers into threads.

Does this sound like instant gratification to you? Hardly! While some of us make clothing from patterns or sew beautiful quilts, few of us would take the time to spin fiber into thread, weave threads into cloth, and then sew the cloth into garments. The Proverbs 31 woman sounds like someone of supreme patience, willing to do whatever is necessary to have things done right and with excellence.

I see her sitting alone in a sunny courtyard, enjoying the solitude, singing a song of praise to God. Or perhaps she's in a circle of friends who are spinning thread as well. She's laughing and enjoying their company as they share a common pursuit.

Whatever you do today, do it with excellence and go the extra mile. You may set your hands to the computer or reach out to shake the hand of a client. Perhaps your hands will wipe the tears of a crying child or clean up a mess you didn't make.

Your words can reach out to others, too. Ask the Lord whom you can touch today with words of kindness and encouragement.

Lord, my prayer today is... "Heavenly Father, I'm grateful that You have made me a woman of excellence, purpose, and vision. I know You have because in these last days, You are calling all of us to believe You for great things to reach a lost and hurting world with the truth that Jesus is the ultimate and only answer. I will extend my hands and my heart today as You guide me. Amen."

‏ Mini-Workout

PraiseMoves Alphabetics: Yod—
The Closed Hand ("Work, a Deed, to Make")

Sitting on the floor, bring your knees to your chest. Bring your forehead toward your knees, wrapping your arms around your knees and grasping your wrist. Breathe gently. For an added challenge, see if you can balance on your tailbone.

Meditate on today's scripture (Proverbs 31:19).

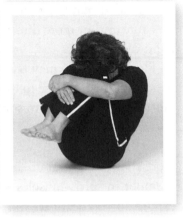

PraiseMoves Workout: The Fisher

Lie on your back with your legs extended and your toes pointed. Place your hands under your hips, palms down. Breathe deeply. Slowly raise yourself onto your elbows, arching your upper back and tilting your head backward. Rest gently on the top of your head before returning to the starting position.

Scripture to meditate on: Jesus said, "Follow Me, and I will make you fishers of men" (Matthew 4:19).

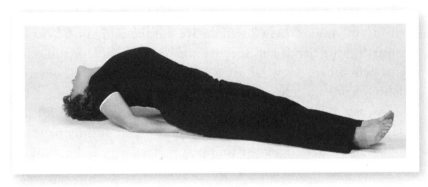

Day 11

Scripture for today. "She opens her hand to the poor, yes, she reaches out her filled hands to the needy [whether in body, mind, or spirit]" (Proverbs 31:20 AMP, brackets in original).

Insights into the Word. It takes wisdom and direction from God to know how to help others in need. While the words "poor" and "needy" seem to describe the same condition, their definitions in Hebrew paint a different picture. The poor one mentioned first may be someone who is feeling sad or depressed. She would benefit from an extended hand of friendship and comfort. The needy person is destitute and in more dire straits. She requires more help than one hand can give her.

Helping people may take extra work on our part. Opening my hand to someone close to me is easier than reaching and stretching out my "filled hands" to someone I may not know as well or even a stranger.

In this instance, the word "hands" *(yadh)* is significant. It means more than the plural of "hand" *(kaf)*. The *hand (kaf)* we open to the poor in spirit consoles and soothes, while the *hands (yadh)* we extend to the destitute must be filled with something greater in order to make a lasting difference. Yes, your hands can be filled with tangible goods to meet the person's immediate needs, but the word *yadh* implies that strength and power also accompany your gift. You're to give more than a mere handout.

We've heard the expression that people need a "hand up" more than just a handout. As Christians we are the body of Christ on this earth. Our hands and feet are the ones available for Him to use to help others. How far are we willing to go to reach out and touch someone for Jesus?

Lord, my prayer today is... "Heavenly Father, I ask You for the wisdom to know how and to whom I'm to reach out my hands. I want to reach out to others in Your power, not my own. I'm limited in what I have to give anyone, but You are unlimited. Please give me the words to say that will make a difference in someone's life today. I also trust You to give me wisdom to know what material gifts would be most meaningful to those people. Help me to be an answer to someone's prayer today. In Jesus' name, amen."

ꓶ *Mini-Workout*
PraiseMoves Alphabetics: Kaf—The Open Hand
("To Open, to Cover, to Allow")

Sitting up straight on the floor, extend your legs in front of you and bring them together, pointing your toes. Hold your abdomen in.

Hinge forward from your hips and reach your hands forward, palms up. Stretch and breathe deeply. Don't lift your head up; maintain a straight line from the crown of your head all the way down your spine.

Meditate on today's scripture (Proverbs 31:20).

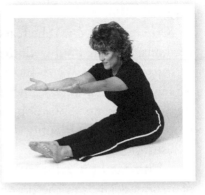

PraiseMoves Workout: Jars of Clay

Sit up straight with your knees bent, feet flat on the floor. Reach under your legs and hold onto the back of your knees. Slowly lean back and lift your legs, balancing on your tailbone if you can. Breathe gently. When you're ready, let go of your legs and straighten them upward into a V-sit, pointing your toes. Reach your arms out in front of you, palms up. Keep your back straight and your neck relaxed. Tighten your abdominals.

Scripture to meditate on: "But we have this treasure in earthen vessels, that the excellence of the power may be of God and not of us" (2 Corinthians 4:7).

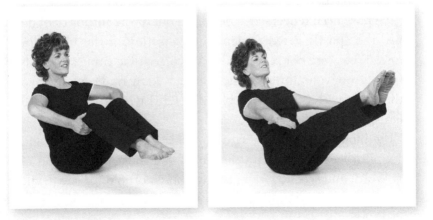

Day 12

Scripture for today. "She fears not the snow for her family, for all her household are doubly clothed in scarlet" (Proverbs 31:21 AMP).

Insights into the Word. Inclement weather will come. Physically we have sweaters, hats, Windbreakers, and galoshes to protect us from the elements. Spiritually we can ensure that our families are protected as well—"doubly clothed in scarlet," the precious blood of Jesus.

In Exodus 12, God instructed the Hebrews to apply the blood of a spotless lamb to the doorposts of their homes for protection. The Lord wouldn't allow the destroyer to take the firstborn of the children of Israel as he would the firstborn of the Egyptians. Death would "pass over" their homes, thus instituting the first Passover, which is celebrated to this day by Jews and some Christians around the world.

By faith you can apply the blood of Jesus to the doorposts of your life and over the lives of your family members.[16] You can apply His blood to any situation with the Bible-inspired words of your mouth. This is what some call "pleading the blood of Jesus." When a judge asks a defendant, "How do you plead?" the person may say "Guilty" or "Innocent." Our answer is, "We are innocent," but not because of our worthiness. Rather, we're saying that the precious blood of Jesus paid the price for our freedom and redemption. He's got us "covered."

We have been redeemed—delivered out of the authority of darkness. The apostle Peter, under the inspiration of the Holy Spirit wrote, "You were not redeemed with corruptible things, like silver or gold, from your aimless conduct received by tradition from your fathers, but with the precious blood of Christ, as of a lamb without blemish and without spot."[17]

The blood of Jesus is a sign of God's covenant—His promise to us. But we must do our part. First, we must believe God and His Word, and second, we must give no "foothold for the devil."[18]

We can then boldly say that our families are not only well clothed physically but spiritually under the blood of Jesus.

Temptations and trials will come. The enemy may form weapons against us, but the Word of the Lord says that if we believe in Him, we shall overcome. Jesus said, "Behold, I give you the authority to trample on serpents and scorpions, and over all the power of the enemy, and nothing shall by any means hurt you."[19] We're "doubly clothed in scarlet."

Lord, my prayer today is… "Heavenly Father, I thank You for covering and protecting me and my family. I place myself in agreement with Your Word, which says, 'No weapon that is formed against you shall prosper, and every tongue that shall rise against you in judgment you shall show to be in the wrong. This [peace, righteousness, security, triumph over opposition] is the heritage of the servants of the Lord [those in whom the ideal Servant of the Lord is reproduced]; this is the righteousness or the vindication which they obtain from Me [this is that which I impart to them as their justification], says the Lord.'"[20] Amen."

ל *Mini-Workout*

PraiseMoves Alphabetics:
Lamed—The Tongue
("Control, Authority, Tongue")

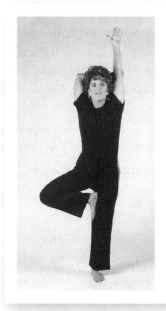

Standing on your left leg, bend your right leg and bring the sole of your right foot to rest against the inside of your left calf or thigh. (Until you build better balance, you may want to place the instep of your right foot over the top of your left foot.) Keep your abdominals tight and your pelvis tucked under. Raise your left arm (the same arm as your standing leg) straight overhead. Bring your right hand behind your head and grasp your left elbow. Lift up straight and tall. Press your bent knee back, opening up the angle of your hip and thigh. Breathe deeply. Release the hold and repeat on the other side.

Meditate on today's scripture (Proverbs 31:21).

PraiseMoves Workout: The Tree

Place the instep of one foot over the top of the other and bend your knees slightly. Keep your abdominals tight and your pelvis tucked under. Inhale slowly, then exhale, lifting your arms overhead like the branches of a tree. Repeat on the other side.

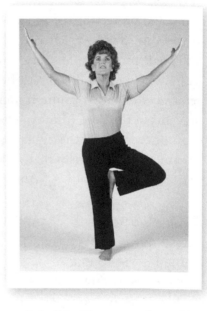

To build balance, place one foot on the inside of your calf or thigh (not the knee). Focus your eyes on one spot in front of you to keep your balance, then reach your arms up. Keep your bent knee pressed back to ensure that your thigh and hip stay at an open angle. Repeat on the other side.

Scriptural affirmation to meditate on: I shall be like a tree planted by the rivers of water, that brings forth its fruit in its season, whose leaf also shall not wither; and whatever I do shall prosper (Psalm 1:3).

Day 13

Scripture for today. "She makes for herself coverlets, cushions, and rugs of tapestry. Her clothing is of linen, pure and fine, and of purple [such as that of which the clothing of the priests and the hallowed cloths of the temple were made]" (Proverbs 31:22 AMP, brackets in original).

Insights into the Word. We can enjoy luxury and surround ourselves with beautiful things (whether we create them or buy them). We can make our homes quiet havens of rest and comfort and wear stylish clothing that looks attractive and modest. The Lord wants us to have nice things; He just doesn't want those nice things to "have" us. They're not to take first place in our lives, thus becoming idols.

Even if we are busy, virtuous women, it's important that we understand the effect the atmosphere we've created has on those we love. We create our environment more with our words and our actions than with fine fabrics and furnishings. The words we say color our homes and lives with love or hatred. We can decorate our homes with praise or complaints, with peace and trust or fear, worry, and suspicion.

We're a royal priesthood; kings and priests[21] of the most high God. As such, we are clothed in righteousness, gladness, and humility.[22] When we're tempted to say ugly things about ourselves, our loved ones, our jobs, or our homes, we can capture those words before they leave our mouths—before they can "decorate" our surroundings.

It's important to take control of our thought lives and dwell on Philippians 4:8 areas instead: "Finally, brethren, whatever things are true, whatever things are noble, whatever things are just, whatever things are pure, whatever things are lovely, whatever things are of good report, if there is any virtue and if there is anything praiseworthy—meditate on these things."

Lord, my prayer today is… "Heavenly Father, I purpose to decorate my home with beauty in thought, word, and deed. Please show me how I can make my environment a place of peace, comfort, and joy—a piece of heaven on earth. Help me to also bring some of that heaven with me wherever I go so that I may be a fit ambassador for You. Amen."

מ *Mini-Workout*
PraiseMoves Alphabetics: Mem—
Water ("Liquid, Massive, Chaos")

Kneel, resting your bottom lightly on your heels. For added comfort, you may want to place a towel or pillow under your knees. Place your hands on the floor behind you, pointing your fingers toward your toes. Gently lift your hips up and tighten your behind. Look up at the ceiling, keeping your neck and shoulders relaxed. Breathe deeply.

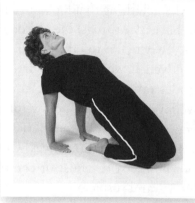

Meditate on today's scripture (Proverbs 31:22).

PraiseMoves Workout: The Little Child

Begin facedown on your abdomen with your legs together. Push your body up into a sitting posture on your haunches, keeping your knees together and underneath you. Slowly bend forward, lowering your body until your forehead is resting on the floor. Move your arms to your sides or overhead and rest them on the floor. Relax your face and neck. To modify this posture, you can sit on a pillow or spread your knees apart if that's more comfortable.

Scripture to meditate on: Jesus said, "Assuredly, I say to you, whoever does not receive the kingdom of God as a little child will by no means enter it" (Mark 10:15).

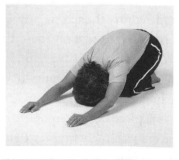

Day 14

Scripture for today. "Her husband is known in the [city's] gates, when he sits among the elders of the land" (Proverbs 31:23 AMP, brackets in original).

Insights into the Word. You have a circle of influence, and if you're married, you and your husband have a circle of influence together as well. You can have an effect on others through your prayers and by taking action as the Lord gives you ideas about how to bless people. We can, like Jabez, ask the Lord to bless (empower) us and "enlarge [our] territory."[23] Your territory can be a physical area, but it can also be the influence you have for good.

Lord, my prayer today is... "Heavenly Father, I ask You to expand the areas of influence of every member of my family and the territories we reach. I pray that we will be blessings to the people You put across our paths and that my family's name will be associated with integrity, excellence, and godliness. I want us to honor the name of Jesus and the title 'Christian.' I pray this in Jesus' name. Amen."

꒕ *Mini-Workout*

PraiseMoves Alphabetics: Nun—
Fish Darting Through Water ("Activity, Life")

Sit up straight with your knees bent, and your feet on the floor, your abdominals tight. Place your feet together, insteps touching, and gently bring your heels toward you. Hold on to your ankles or feet and see if you can very gently lower your knees to the floor. You can press them lightly downward with your elbows or hands. Breathe deeply.

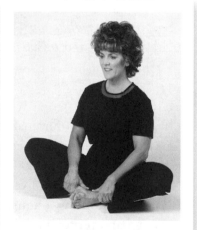

Keep your back as straight as possible and your head in a neutral position.

Meditate on today's scripture (Proverbs 31:23).

PraiseMoves Workout: The Turn-Away Twist

Sit on the floor with both legs out in front of you. Bend your right knee, lift your right leg over your left, and place your right foot on the floor next to your left knee. Sitting with your spine straight, gently pull your bent knee with your opposite hand. Place your right hand on the floor behind you for support. Lower your left arm, touching your right hip with your left fingertips while gently twisting to look over your right shoulder. Be careful not to twist too far. Hold for a few seconds, release, and repeat on 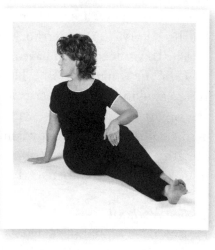 the opposite side (bending your left knee and placing your left leg over your right, etc.).

Scripture to meditate on: "Turn away my eyes from looking at worthless things, and revive me in Your way" (Psalm 119:37).

Day 15

Scripture for today. "She makes fine linen garments and leads others to buy them; she delivers to the merchants girdles [or sashes that free one up for service]" (Proverbs 31:24 AMP, brackets in original).

Insights into the Word. Every woman works, whether she works at a business, running a home, or both. In this age of technology, it's easier than ever for women to do both, and some choose to do so while working in the comfort of their homes.

The Amplified Version paints a picture of a successful home-based woman entrepreneur: She "leads others to buy." She doesn't manipulate anyone to do anything. Unfortunately, we've all had that unpleasant experience of feeling pressured to buy something. The Lord is also One who leads and guides us. He never forces us. But the enemy pushes us, saying, "You've got to do it now. Buy it now. Have it now! Hurry, hurry, hurry!"

When we have something of value we want to tell people about, whether it's a product we believe in or our Lord and Savior Jesus Christ, we can lead and guide them by sharing the truth in love with enthusiasm and integrity. I imagine the virtuous woman telling her friends how *she* feels wearing linen and how much she enjoys the garments. No one can argue with your personal testimony.

Lord, my prayer today is… "Heavenly Father, help me share the gifts and talents You've given me with those around me. Your Word says that my 'gift makes room for [me] and brings [me] before great men [and women].'[24] Thank You for enabling me to do all You call me to do. Amen."

◌ Mini-Workout
PraiseMoves Alphabetics: Samech—Support
("Support, Twist Slowly, Turn")

Lie down on your abdomen with your forehead on the mat and your legs extended. Place your arms at your sides, palms up. Slowly raise your head, arms, and legs at the same time. Look up toward the ceiling. To modify this pos-ture, keep your hands on the floor at your sides, palms down or make fists. If you'd like more of a challenge, reach back, grasp one or both ankles, and lift up slowly, looking at the ceiling. In PraiseMoves this posture is called "Peter's Boat."

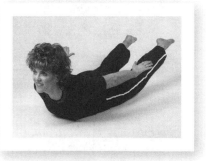

Meditate on today's scripture (Proverbs 31:24).

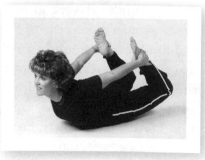

Slow-Cadence Exercise: Push-Ups

Start in a push-up position with your hands directly under your shoulders, your arms straight (but not locked), and your legs extended. (If a classic push-up is too difficult for you right now, start on your knees until you build up enough upper-body strength.) Keep your back straight and your abdomen tight. Tuck in your chin slightly to avoid craning or injuring your neck. Inhale and slowly lower your body to the floor to a count of 8. Pause briefly when your chest touches the floor, then exhale as you push back up at the very slow count of 8. Don't rest at the bottom of the motion; immediately begin to push back up to the starting position. Don't lock your elbows when you reach the top. Breathe gently, and don't hold your breath or contort your face.

Continue with proper form for 2 minutes or until muscle failure.

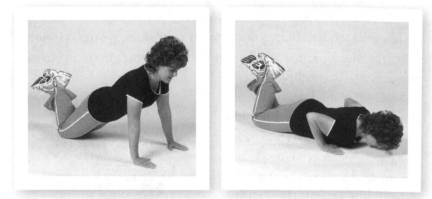

Scripture to meditate on: "I press toward the goal for the prize of the upward call of God in Christ Jesus" (Philippians 3:14).

Day 16

Scripture for today. "Strength and dignity are her clothing and her position is strong and secure; she rejoices over the future [the latter day or time to come, knowing that she and her family are in readiness for it]" (Proverbs 31:25 AMP, brackets in original).

Insights into the Word. When strength and dignity are your clothing, you're a "power dresser" no matter *what* you wear! We can "be strong in the Lord and in the power of His might."[25] Our faith in the almighty nature of God makes us secure in the knowledge that our strength is in Him. He won't waver, falter, or fail. We can come off our foundation, but our foundation will never move. We can remain secure by staying in fellowship with the Lord and standing on His Word.

Have you rejoiced over your future lately? That's not something many of us think of doing. Like everything else we do as believers, it requires trusting the Lord in spite of how things may appear. Having a relationship with Him ensures our eternal future—and we can rejoice in our immediate future as well—no matter what!

God said through the prophet Jeremiah, "For I know the thoughts that I think toward you, says the LORD, thoughts of peace and not of evil, to give you a future and a hope."[26] His thoughts and plans for us are all for good, and by being attentive to the inner leading of His Spirit, we can be prepared for any adjustments we need to make along the way. We usually know when something we've planned to do just doesn't feel right...even if it seems the logical choice. The Lord's leading is subtle, by His "still small voice."[27] We can trust His guidance in our lives, so rejoice!

Lord, my prayer today is... "Heavenly Father, thank You for clothing me in strength and dignity. You are the strength of my life. I'm grateful that You lead and guide me, and I rejoice that my future and my family's future are secure in You. I'm becoming more sensitive to Your leading every day. Thank You for helping us prepare for the days ahead. I praise and worship You! Amen."

ב *Mini-Workout*
PraiseMoves Alphabetics:
Ayin—The Eye ("To See, to
Know, to Experience")

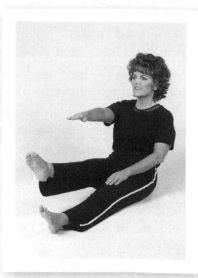

Sit up straight on the floor with your legs out in front of you. Slowly raise your right leg and right arm at the same time. Keep your palm facing down and point your toes. Keep your back straight and your abdominals tight. Breathe gently. Switch to your left leg and arm and repeat.

Meditate on today's scripture (Proverbs 31:25).

PraiseMoves Posture:
The Table

Sit on the floor with your knees bent, your feet on the floor, and your hands behind you, fingertips pointing toward your heels. Tighten your abdominals. Push up until your torso is straight across, like a table. Keep your head in neutral position and look at the ceiling. Breathe gently. Extend one leg, hold, then bring it back. Repeat with the other leg.

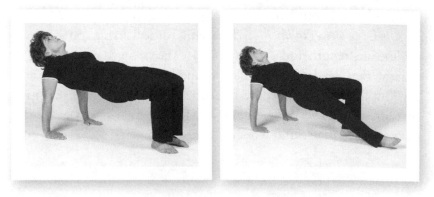

Scripture to meditate on: "You prepare a table before me in the presence of my enemies" (Psalm 23:5).

Day 17

Scripture for today. "She opens her mouth in skillful and godly Wisdom, and on her tongue is the law of kindness [giving counsel and instruction]" (Proverbs 31:26 AMP, brackets in original).

Insights into the Word. The only way "skillful and godly Wisdom" can come out of our mouths is if it's deposited in our hearts. Jesus said, "Out of the abundance of the heart the mouth speaks."[28] Whatever there is in abundance in our hearts is what will come out of our mouths.

We want to share the "skillful and godly Wisdom" with kindness—"speaking the truth in love," not judgment.[29] But what if we don't know what to say? Thankfully, we can ask the Lord for the words to say in any situation, and He will guide us! In Psalm 81:10 He says, "Open your mouth wide, and I will fill it."

Many times we have to be willing to open our mouths in faith before all the words come. Sometimes I'm given a scripture or just a few words of encouragement to share with someone. However, once I begin sharing what the Lord has placed on my heart, the rest follows. He is faithful to His Word and to us.

Lord, my prayer today is... "Heavenly Father, I purpose to fill my heart, mind, and mouth with Your thoughts and words. I can be sure I'm operating more and more in 'godly Wisdom' when I meditate on and speak Your Word. Thank You in advance for enabling me to use Your words skillfully, with kindness and love, so I may be a blessing in the lives of others. Amen."

⌐ *Mini-Workout*
PraiseMoves Alphabetics: Pe—The Mouth
("To Speak, a Word, to Open")

Get down on your knees and place your hands on your hips, fingers pointing forward. Tighten your abdominals and glutes.

Slowly lean back several inches, feeling a stretch in the quads (front of your thighs). Look up toward the ceiling. Breathe gently. Return to starting position.

Meditate on today's scripture (Proverbs 31:26).

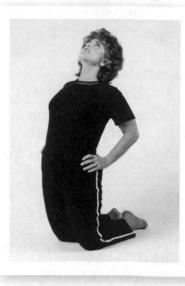

Slow-Cadence Exercise: Abdominal Crunches

Lie on your back with your knees bent and your feet flat on the floor. Place your fingers behind your head and your thumbs by your temples or jaw. You'll lift up using only your abdominal muscles. Do *not* jerk your neck up. Keep your head cradled in your hands, elbows out to the sides. Push your lower back into the floor and look up at the ceiling as you slowly lift your chest and shoulders off the floor to a count of 8. Keep your head in the same position, cradled in your hands, while looking straight up at the ceiling (not forward).

When you reach the top of the lift, squeeze your abdominal muscles for a moment and then slowly lower back to the floor to a count of 8. Breathe gently and evenly throughout the exercise, and keep your face relaxed.

Add the scripture when you're comfortable with the exercise and are sure you're maintaining the proper form.

Scriptural affirmation to meditate on: I lay aside every weight and the sin

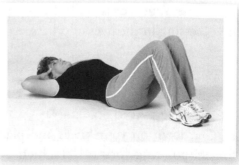

which so easily ensnares me, and I run with endurance the race that is set before me, looking unto Jesus, the author and finisher of my faith (Hebrews 12:1-2).

Day 18

Scripture for today. "She looks well to how things go in her household, and the bread of idleness (gossip, discontent, and self-pity) she will not eat" (Proverbs 31:27 AMP).

Insights into the Word. "Idleness" is defined in the Amplified Version as "gossip, discontent, and self-pity." Many of us thought idleness was standing around doing nothing (which we busy women *never* do!). Actually, the verse says "she *will not* eat" the "bread of idleness," so it seems to be something we determine we will or won't do.

Have you ever been invited to attend a gossip session or hold your own pity party? Our carnal nature delights in these diversions. One thing we can begin doing to resist these temptations is to speak good things over the various households we occupy: our families and homes, our church bodies (the "household of faith"), and our physical bodies (the "home" in which we live). Instead of tearing down these households by engaging in what is wrong ("gossip, discontent, and self-pity"), we can build them up by focusing on what is right and thanking God for them.

Lord, my prayer today is… "Heavenly Father, thank You for helping me order my priorities to do what is mine to do today. I purpose to see the good in others in order to encourage them and call them up higher in their relationship with the Lord. I say with the psalmist David, 'Set a guard, O LORD, over my mouth; keep watch over the door of my lips'[30] and 'Let the words of my mouth and the meditation of my heart be acceptable in Your sight, O LORD, my strength and my Redeemer.'[31] Amen."

⅏ *Mini-Workout*

PraiseMoves Alphabetics:
Tsadde—The Fish Hook
("Catch, Desire, Need")

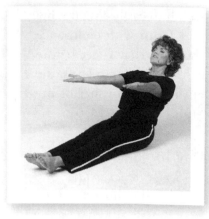

Sit up straight with your legs out in front of you. Tighten your abdominals. Raise your arms and hands, palms up, and slowly lean back as far as you comfortable can to work the abdominals. For more of a challenge, you can raise your legs slightly. Breathe gently and evenly; don't hold your breath!

Meditate on today's scripture (Proverbs 31:27).

PraiseMoves Workout: The Scroll

Sit up straight with your legs out in front of you. Place your hands on the top of your thighs, then fold over your legs, keeping your back straight and your abdominals tight. Look up at the ceiling until you've come as far as you comfortably can. Let your head and neck relax and your torso go limp over your legs. Breathe gently and deeply. With each exhalation, see if you can go just one millimeter deeper into the stretch.

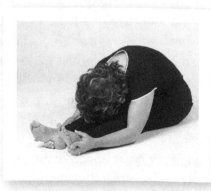

Slowly round your body up to the starting position. Repeat the stretch with one leg out in front of you and the opposite leg bent, with your foot pressed into your thigh. Hold for a few breaths, then switch legs and repeat. Finally, with both legs comfortably apart (in a V), gently walk your hands along the floor in front of you. Relax and then put your weight on your hands as you slowly round back up to the starting position.

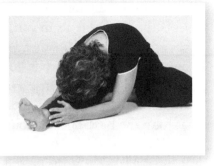

Scripture to meditate on: "As His custom was, [Jesus] went into the synagogue on the Sabbath day, and stood up to read. And He was handed the book of the prophet Isaiah. And when He had opened the book, He found the place where it was written: 'The Spirit of the Lord is upon Me, because He has anointed Me to preach the gospel to the poor'" (Luke 4:16-18).

Day 19

Scripture for today. "Her children rise up and call her blessed (happy, fortunate, and to be envied); and her husband boasts of and praises her, [saying], 'Many daughters have done virtuously, nobly, and well [with the strength of character that is steadfast in goodness], but you excel them all'" (Proverbs 31:28-29 AMP, brackets in original).

Insights into the Word. Over the years, today's verses have been prayed by countless women whose children have risen up and called them everything except "blessed" and whose husbands seem to be more at home on the range, "where seldom is heard an encouraging word." But in time, many of these women have seen God's promise in these verses come to pass.

How do others see you? Can you imagine being called blessed, virtuous, noble, and of a strong, godly character? Do you see yourself that way? If not, why not? Well, you aren't capable of drumming up these qualities yourself—no human is. But God is the Source of "every good and perfect gift,"[32] so you can ask Him to work them through you as you yield to the fruit of the Spirit ("love, joy, peace, patience, kindness, goodness, faithfulness, gentleness, and self-control").[33] Doing so will produce the godly character that causes others to see Jesus in you. Then when others call you blessed, virtuous, or good, you can give all the credit and glory to God, knowing it was certainly His doing, not your own.

Lord, my prayer today is... "Heavenly Father, I want people to see Your goodness in me, to see more of You and less of me. I will say what John the Baptist said about You, Lord: '[You] must increase, but I must decrease.'[34] Help me be the person You have called me to be. I pray that my family and others will see Jesus in me so they will be drawn to You. Amen."

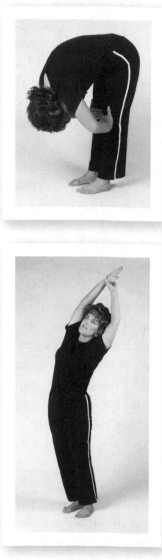

Mini-Workout (Two Letters Today!)

ק PraiseMoves Alphabetics: Kuf— The Back of the Head ("Behind, the Last, the Least")

Start in a standing position. Bend forward, rounding your back and placing your hands above your knees, with your fingers pointing toward each other. Press your elbows toward the floor. Keep your knees straight (but not locked) and your abdominals tight. Breathe gently and evenly.

Meditate on today's scripture (Proverbs 31:28).

ר PraiseMoves Alphabetics: Resh— The Head of a Man ("A Person, the Head, the Highest")

Stand with your feet together, reaching both arms overhead with your palms facing each other. Slowly lift up through your waist and bend slightly to the right. Breathe deeply. For an added stretch, gently grasp your left wrist with your right hand. Keep your pelvis tucked under and your abdominals tight to protect your lower back. Lower your arms and repeat on the other side.

Meditate on today's scripture (Proverbs 31:29).

PraiseMoves Workout: The Angel

Bring one leg behind you, heel to the floor. Bend the knee of the leg in front so that your knee aligns with your ankle. Keep your abdominals tight. Breathe gently. Raise your arms overhead and slowly stretch from your hips and waist all the way up through your fingertips. If you can, bring your upper arms alongside your ears. Look forward and down slightly, keeping your head in a neutral position. If you want to work on balance, slowly lift your back leg behind you up bit by bit. Find a point to focus on as you build balance. Repeat on the other side.

Scripture to meditate on: "He shall give His angels charge over you, to keep you in all your ways" (Psalm 91:11).

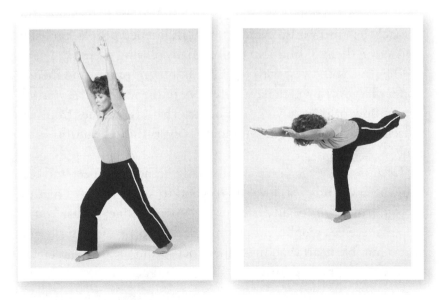

Day 20

Scripture for today. "Charm and grace are deceptive, and beauty is vain [because it is not lasting], but a woman who reverently and worshipfully fears the Lord, she shall be praised!" (Proverbs 31:30 AMP, brackets in original).

Insights into the Word. "The things which are seen are temporary, but the things which are not seen are eternal."[35] While charm and poise may seem appealing in "polite" company, these qualities can be fleeting and mercurial. They may also not be accurate indicators of the real person.

We've all seen videos on the news of famous people who, while normally composed and polite, have lost all charm and grace when their tempers got the better of them. Gratefully, most of us don't have to worry about our every foible being broadcast on the nightly news. People *are* watching us, however. Our neighbors, unsaved loved ones, coworkers, and our immediate families are watching and learning from us.

The good news is that the work we allow the Lord to do on the inside of us has a way of showing in our lives and in our countenances. When Moses came down from the mountain after spending time in God's presence for 40 days and nights, his face shone. The glory of the Lord was so evident that it frightened people (probably convicting them of sin more than actually scaring them).[36]

The time you invest with the Lord in prayer, praise, and meditation on His Word will make a difference in the way you see yourself and in how others see you. The beauty that lasts comes from the reflected glory of the One who makes "everything beautiful in its time."[37]

Lord, my prayer today is... "Heavenly Father, I respect and fear You with awe and great love. It's so good to know that as I mature in You, real *lasting* beauty is being developed in me. I trust You to help me receive compliments and praise from others graciously and with a humble heart that draws their focus from me to You. You are worthy of all praise! Amen."

♙ *Mini-Workout*

PraiseMoves Alphabetics:
Shin—The Teeth ("To
Consume, to Destroy")

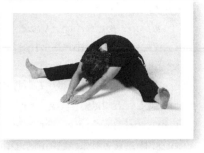

Sit with your legs wide apart and your hands on the floor in front of you. Keeping your back as straight as possible and your abdominals tight, slowly walk your hands forward along the floor, lowering your head and torso. Relax and breathe gently. To come out of the posture, put your weight on your hands and walk back up to a straight-back position.

Meditate on today's scripture (Proverbs 31:30).

PraiseMoves Workout: Rest and Stretch

Lie on your back with your knees bent and your feet flat on the floor. Slide your arms out to the sides in line with your shoulders,

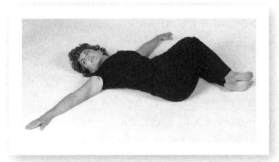

palms down, keeping contact with the floor. Lower your knees to the right, and turn your head to the left, breathing gently. Return to center, then repeat on the other side.

Next, bring your knees toward your chest, and follow the same sequence.

Scripture to meditate on: Jesus said, "Come to Me, all you who labor and are heavy laden, and I will give you rest" (Matthew 11:28).

Day 21

Scripture for today. "Give her of the fruit of her hands, and let her own works praise her in the gates [of the city]!" (Proverbs 31:31 AMP, brackets in original).

Insights into the Word. The fruit of your hands represents the results of your labor. You're rewarded for your work in various ways. If you work at a business, you expect to be compensated for your efforts. But rewards are more than financial. It's good to know you're doing the work the Lord has called you to do using the gifts and talents He's given you. Making a positive difference in the lives of others is also a blessing. Committing your day and your work to the Lord and being sensitive to His leading will help ensure that you're following Him.

In Bible times the city gates were where business was conducted and legal matters were decided by the elders. As Proverbs tells us, people were praised for their works at the city gates as well. Few cities have gates today, but you can still be known in your community as a person of honesty and integrity. The key is following this verse from Colossians: "Whatever you do, do it heartily, as to the Lord and not to men, knowing that from the Lord you will receive the reward of the inheritance; for you serve the Lord Christ."[38]

Lord, my prayer today is… "Heavenly Father, help me be sensitive to Your leading as I follow You today. I purpose to do everything You call me to do to the best of my ability. I won't look to people for promotion and acceptance, but to You, knowing that my ultimate purpose in life is to serve You in all I do. Amen."

♫ *Mini-Workout*

PraiseMoves Alphabetics: Tav—The Cross

("To Seal, to Covenant")

Modified Cross: Come down onto all fours with your hands directly under your shoulders, your fingers spread apart. Straighten one leg behind you, then the other, bringing your body into a straight line and keeping your toes in contact with the floor. Tighten your abdominals and keep your head in a neutral position. This is the altar position.

Bend your right knee, keeping your left leg extended. Place your weight on the bent knee and your right hand as you slowly turn your body toward the left, bringing your left hand up, palm facing forward. Keep your right arm straight (but not locked). Your arms should be in the shape of a cross. Breathe gently and evenly. Repeat on the other side.

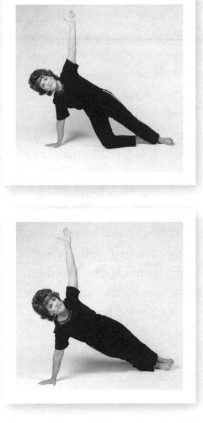

After you feel comfortable with your performance of the modified Cross, try the advanced Cross: Return to The Altar posture. Place your weight on your right hand as you turn to bring the soles of your feet together. If this is too difficult at first, place one foot in front of the other for balance. When you have your balance, slowly lift your top arm toward the ceiling to form a cross, with your palm facing forward.

Meditate on today's scripture (Proverbs 31:31).

PraiseMoves Workout: The Tent

Get on your hands and knees, with your toes contacting the floor underneath you (not pointing), legs hip-width apart, and arms shoulder-width apart and a foot in front of you. Spread your fingers wide apart, with your middle fingers parallel to each other, pointing straight ahead. Rotate the inside of your elbows forward. With your arms straight (but not locked), slowly raise your hips up and back, reaching your tailbone toward the ceiling and straightening your legs. Keep your head in a neutral position. Press your heels toward the floor for an added calf stretch. You can bend your knees slightly to help straighten your back. Remember to breathe gently throughout the exercise. Bend your knees to come out of "The Tent" and come back down to the original posture.

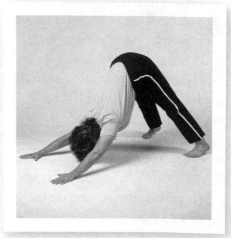

Scripture to meditate on: "Enlarge the place of your tent, and let them stretch out the curtains of your dwellings; do not spare; lengthen your cords, and strengthen your stakes" (Isaiah 54:2).

MAKING IT PERSONAL

1. Something I learned about the Lord during these daily studies
   is: _____
   _____

2. An answer to prayer I received is: _____
   _____
   _____
   _____

3. Several positive habits I've developed over the last few weeks I
   want to continue are: _____
   _____
   _____
   _____
   _____

CONGRATULATIONS AND KEEP GOING!

Set a New Goal

Congratulations on sticking with this book and program! How did you do in the past three weeks on reaching your Total Fitness goals? Did you do as well as you wanted to do? Did you surprise yourself in some areas and learn new things about yourself?

This book is about Total Fitness, which includes physical fitness and the well-being of your spirit and soul. All three are important! If you learned even one new thing these last few weeks—if you implemented one change or began to do something differently—you're making progress. Don't be hard on yourself if you didn't excel as much as you wanted. More importantly, don't listen to the enemy's lies that "You blew it!" or some such nonsense. You're still here, so you're up for the journey.

As you reflect on your Total Fitness journey, take out a notebook, journal, or use the "Making It Personal" section to set some new goals for yourself in the coming days and weeks. Be realistic but dare to dream big, too! Write down small steps you can take today and tomorrow and the next day that will lead you to accomplish the goals you and the Lord set and work on together. Remember, "[You] can do all things through Christ who strengthens [you]"![1]

MAKING IT PERSONAL

1. Several new goals I plan for myself are...

Spiritual: _____
_____
_____
_____

Emotional/Mental: _____
_____
_____
_____

Physical: _____
_____
_____
_____

Social/Relationships: _____
_____
_____
_____

Financial/Work-related: _____
_____
_____
_____

Other: _____
_____
_____

2. I believe the Lord is leading me to trust Him more in: _____

_____

_____

_____

3. I purpose to follow the Lord more closely by doing these things on a more consistent basis: _____

_____

_____

_____

_____

4. Instead of falling prey to doubt or worry, I will remember to:

_____

_____

_____

_____

_____

A SPECIAL INVITATION

If you've never received God's gift of salvation through faith in His Son Jesus Christ, you can begin a new life in Him today. God loves you so much and wants to come into your life to change you from the inside out. He died on the cross to reconcile you to God, and then He was raised to life so you can have eternal life in Him. Knowing and following Him will change your life in great, amazing ways. And it will transform your journey toward Total Fitness! Ask Jesus to be your Lord and Savior by praying this prayer:

> Dear God in heaven,
>
> I come to You in the name of Your Son Jesus. Your Word says that "Whoever calls on the name of the LORD shall be saved" and made whole.[1] So I know You want to take me in, and I thank You for it.
>
> Your Word also says, "If you confess with your mouth the Lord Jesus and believe in your heart that God has raised Him from the dead, you will be saved....For whoever calls on the name of the LORD shall be saved."[2]

I believe in my heart that Jesus is the Son of God. I believe He died on the cross to pay for my sins. I believe He was raised from the dead by God's power. I confess out loud with my mouth that Jesus is Lord. I am calling right now on the name of the Lord—on the name of Jesus—so I know I'm saved. Thank You for making it so very simple to receive everlasting life from You right this moment!

I'm now a Christian, and Jesus is living in my heart by the Holy Spirit!

Thank You, heavenly Father! Amen.

Signed: _____

Date: _____

Action Steps for the New Christian

Now that you've accepted Jesus Christ as your Lord and Savior, you're part of the family of God—the body of Christ! Here are a few action steps to help you grow in your faith and walk with Jesus every day!

1. Go to a Bible-believing church. Church is where you learn how to live the Christian life and where the pastor, spiritual leaders, and Christian friends can help you and encourage your faith.

2. Ask to be baptized in water in obedience to the Word of God (see Matthew 28:19; Mark 16:16; Acts 2:38).

3. Read your Bible every day. Start with the Gospel of John. Get a version of the Bible you can understand and ask the Holy Spirit to reveal the truth and power of God's Word to you. (The Bible tells us that the Holy Spirit is our Teacher ["He will teach you all things" (John 14:26)] and "Comforter" [John 14:16,26 KJV]. Now He lives in your heart!)

4. Pray every day. Don't worry about using fancy words or formal language. Simply speak from your heart to your Father God and fellowship with Him. He will hear your prayers and give you the guidance and help you need. He doesn't always answer our prayers the way we expect Him to or in our timing, but He's always faithful to His Word, and He will answer.

5. Strive to live a holy life—a life set apart to God. You aren't perfect—and neither is anyone else. With the Holy Spirit living in us, we can, however, turn from our old, sinful ways and seek to live a life pleasing to God and in accordance with His guidelines set forth in the Bible.

ANSWERS TO "MAKING IT PERSONAL" EXERCISES

Chapter 1—Fitness for the Spirit, Soul, and Body = Total Fitness

1. I am a *spirit*. I have a *soul* and live in a *body*.

2. Answers from personal experience.

3. Romans 14:23 says, "Whatever is not from faith is sin." Answer to second question from your personal experience.

4. Answers from personal experience.

5. Answers from personal experience.

Chapter 2—Quick Nutrition Tips

1–4. Answers from personal experience.

Chapter 3—The Best Miracle Elixir for the Money

1. *More than half* of my body is made up of water.

2. How much water should I drink each day? A good rule of thumb is half my *body weight* in ounces.

3. Chronic dehydration can lead to a host of debilitating conditions, including *neck and back pain, arthritis and other kinds of joint pain, kidney stones,* and *high blood pressure.*

4–6. Answers from personal experience.

Chapter 4—Quick and Safe Weight-Loss Tips

1. God said in Deuteronomy 30:19, "I call heaven and earth as witnesses today against you, that I have set before you *life* and *death,* blessing and cursing; therefore choose *life,* that both you and your descendants may live."

2. Answer from personal experience.

3. Include lean protein in *three* meals and *two* snacks.

4. Examples of lean-protein meat sources include hormone-free *chicken and turkey breast, lean grass-fed beef, and fish.* Nonmeat sources include *soy, nuts, eggs and low-fat dairy products,* and *vegetable-protein products.*

5. It's important that you don't go for more than *three* hours without something to eat in order to avoid the starvation response.

6. Portion sizes are important. A portion (one serving) is about the size of a *deck* of *cards.*

7. Answer from personal experience.

Chapter 5—Your Fitness Personality

1–4. Answers from personal experience.

Chapter 6—Fitness for the Busy Woman

1–4. Answers from personal experience.

Chapter 7—Breathing—Escape the Shallows

1. *Oxygen* is the most vital nutrient for our body's survival. We can go for weeks without *food,* days without *water,* but only a few minutes without *oxygen.*

2. Benefits of deep breathing include any of the following: increased energy, reduced mental and physical fatigue, elimination of toxins, improved circulation, endurance, clearer complexion, sound sleep, relief from tension, and more!

3–4. Answers from your own personal experience.

Chapter 8—20 Minutes to Be Fit for the King

1. According to a study in the *American Journal of Clinical Nutrition*, "Although *30* minutes of daily, moderate-intensity physical activity may result in significant improvements in health, it appears that progressing to at least *60* minutes of physical activity may be necessary for enhancing long-term weight loss outcomes."

2. Two ways we may strengthen the fruit of the Spirit in our lives is by *yielding* to the Holy Spirit and His fruit and by *sowing* seeds of patience, faithfulness, self-control (or love, joy, peace, kindness, goodness, and gentleness).

3–4. Answers from your own personal experience.

Chapter 9—PraiseMoves®—The Christian Alternative to Yoga

1. In the words of many Christians and Hindus, including Hindu yoga professor Subhas Tiwari quoted in *Time* magazine, "Yoga is *Hinduism*."

2. Yoga postures are actually *offerings* to 330 million Hindu gods.

3. Acts 15:29 tells us to "abstain from *things* offered to idols."

4. Answer from personal experience with accompanying scripture and reference.

Chapter 10—21 Days to Total Fitness with the Virtuous ("Mighty") Woman

1–4. Answers from your own personal experience.

Congratulations and Keep Going!

1–4. Answers from your own personal experience.

RESOURCES

Please visit www.PraiseMoves.com for information about Praise-Moves classes and DVDs, the Teacher Certification program and instructors in your area, as well as other programs (such as Praise-Moves® for Children, the Gimme Ten Workout, the Slow-Cadence Exercise™ (SCE), QuickFits™, the WOW Workout™, and Praise-Moves® Alphabetics, and others). Check out the PraiseFast program, a spiritual approach to lasting weight loss. Along with the program we have PraiseFast Meal Replacement Shakes and PraiseFast Super Greens.

My website also has resources and additional information on the Hebrew word pictures presented in chapter 10.

In the war against childhood obesity, Laurette has developed a program for public schools called The PowerMoves Kids Program. Designed for K–8th grades, it is the *first* program to combine Character Education and Fitness *in the classroom*. See www.Power MovesKids.com for more information.

If you would like Laurette to visit your church, women's conference, school, or community organization for a Fitness for His Witness Seminar, PraiseMoves® workshop, keynote address, PowerMoves Kids seminar, or one of her one-woman shows (such as "Great Women of the Bible"), please visit www.LauretteWillis.com or e-mail her at Laurette@PraiseMoves.com.

NOTES

We're All Busy

1. "Seek first the kingdom of God and His righteousness, and all these things shall be added to you" (Matthew 6:33).
2. Matthew 25:21.
3. Twelve-step recovery programs are patterned after Alcoholics Anonymous and include such groups as Overeaters Anonymous, Emotions Anonymous, and Narcotics Anonymous. Although the 12 steps of recovery had their roots in the Bible, few programs ascribe to scriptural principles today. One successful Christian program is Celebrate Recovery, which holds meetings at many churches throughout North America and several other countries. (See www.celebrate recovery.com.) Other Christian 12-step programs include Alcoholics Victorious and Overcomers Outreach.
4. Galatians 5:1.
5. For more information about Celebrate Recovery, visit www.celebraterecovery.com.

Chapter 1—Fitness for the Spirit, Soul, and Body = Total Fitness

1. Acts 16:25-26.
2. Galatians 5:1.
3. Hebrews 4:15 NIV.
4. Psalm 56:8; Isaiah 49:16.
5. Exodus 15:26.
6. Ephesians 1:6.
7. Second Corinthians 5:17 says, "Therefore, if anyone is in Christ, he is a new creation; old things have passed away; behold, all things have become new."
8. See Psalm 37:5; Proverbs 3:6; 16:9.
9. Romans 12:2 NLT.
10. Romans 14:23.
11. Romans 10:17.
12. 2 Corinthians 10:5.
13. Paraphrased from Philippians 4:13; Ephesians 6:10; Romans 8:37.

14. Galatians 5:22-23 NLT.

15. "Now the works of the flesh are evident, which are: adultery, fornication, uncleanness, lewdness, idolatry, sorcery, hatred, contentions, jealousies, outbursts of wrath, selfish ambitions, dissensions, heresies, envy, murders, drunkenness, revelries, and the like; of which I tell you beforehand, just as I also told you in time past, that those who practice such things will not inherit the kingdom of God" (Galatians 5:19-21).

Chapter 2—Quick Nutrition Tips

1. Nancy Appleton, "Seventy-Six Ways Sugar Can Ruin Your Health," www. mercola.com/article/sugar/dangers_of_sugar.htm. Information compiled from multiple sources. To see the full list visit Dr. Joseph Mercola's Web site (www. mercola.com/article/sugar/dangers_of_sugar.htm) or read Dr. Appleton's book *Lick the Sugar Habit* (New York: Avery Publishing Group, 1996). This book is available on Dr. Mercola's informative Web site, along with hundreds of other health-related articles.

2. J.O. Hill, et al., "The Role of Breakfast in the Treatment of Obesity," *American Journal of Clinical Nutrition,* 55, no. 3 (Merck 1992): 645-51.

Chapter 3—The Best Miracle Elixir for the Money

1. Research conducted by the NDP Group, cited in John Schmeltzer, "Pop Fans Pour It On in the Morning," *Chicago Tribune,* January 15, 2007, http://www. chicagotribune.com/business/chi0701150103jan15,1,5052844.story?ctrack=1&cs et=true, accessed February 1, 2007.

2. Ibid.

3. "One Sweet Nation," Health: In Brief, *U. S. News and World Report,* March 28, 2005, http://health.usnews.com/usnews/health/articles/050328/28sugar.b.htm, accessed July 7, 2007.

4. Terry L. Davidson and Susan E. Swithers, "A Pavlovian Approach to the Problem of Obesity," *International Journal of Obesity,* 28, no. 77 (July 2004):933-35.

5. David S. Ludwig, Karen E. Peterson, and Steven L. Gortmaker, "Relation Between Consumption of Sugar-Sweetened Drinks and Childhood Obesity: A Prospective, Observational Analysis," *Lancet,* 357, no. 9255 (February 17, 2001):505-08.

6. Ira Bergheim, et al., "Effect of Sugar-Sweetened Beverages on Hepatic Steatosis in Mice," *Hepatology,* 44 (2006), https://www.aasld.org/eweb/dynamicpage. aspx?site=aasld3&webcode=06_pr_damagebysugars, accessed February 1, 2007.

7. Kiejzers, et al., "Caffeine Linked to Diabetes," *Diabetes Care,* 25 (February 2002):364-69, cited in Joseph Mercola, http://cmsadmin.mercola.com/2002/ mar/6/caffeine_diabetes.htm, accessed July 6, 2007.

8. Lars Lien, et al., "Consumption of Soft Drinks and Hyperactivity, Mental Distress, and Conduct Problems Among Adolescents in Oslo, Norway," *American*

Journal of Public Health, 96, no. 10 (October 2006):1815-20, http://www.ncbi. nlm.nih.gov/sites/entrez?cmd=Retrieve&db=PubMed&list_uids=17008578&do pt=Abstract, accessed July 6, 2007.

9. Chris Mercer, "New Benzene Test Reveals Flaw in FDA Soft Drinks Investigation," BeverageDaily.com, April 19, 2006, http://www.beveragedaily. com/news/ng.asp?n=67151-benzene-soft-drinks-fda, accessed February 1, 2007.

10. Nancy Humphrey, "Coffee Institute Receives Kraft Gift," *The Reporter,* Vanderbilt Medical Center, April 27, 2001, http://www.mc.vanderbilt.edu/ reporter/index.html?ID=1487, accessed June 26, 2007.

11. Associated Press, "Two Groups Say Many Drink Unsafe Drinking Water," *New York Times,* June 2, 1995, http://query.nytimes.com/gst/fullpage.html?res=9A06 EFDD1639F931A35755C0A963958260, accessed February 12, 2007.

Chapter 4—Quick and Safe Weight-Loss Tips

1. See John 6:63.

2. John 10:27.

3. Matthew 7:13-14.

4. Proverbs 25:28 niv.

5. Ephesians 5:1.

6. F. Vallejo and R. Puuppoponen-Pimia, news release, *Journal of the Science of Food and Agriculture,* November 2003, vol. 83, 1511-1516, 1389-1402, cited in Jennifer Warren, "Hot Water Kills Broccoli's Benefits," www.webmd.com/food-recipes/news/20031029/hot-water-kills-broccoli, accessed July 29, 2007.

7. Bernard H. Blanc and Hans U. Hertel, "Comparative Study of Food Prepared Conventionally and in the Microwave Oven," *Raum and Zeit* (1992), in *Journal of the Science of Food and Agriculture* 3, no. 2 (November 2003):43. Also see Anthony Wayne and Lawrence Newell, "The Hidden Dangers of Microwave Cooking," www.mercola.com/article/microwave/hazards.htm, accessed July 29, 2007.

8. U.S. Department of Agriculture, "Profiling Food Consumption in America," *Agriculture Fact Book 2001–2002* (Washington D.C.: Government Printing Office, 2002), ch. 2, www.usda.gov/factbook/chapter2.htm.

9. Dianne Neumark-Sztainer, et al., "Are Family Meal Patterns Associated with Disordered Eating Behaviors Among Adolescents?" *Journal of Adolescent Health,* 35, no. 5 (November 2004):350-59, in University of Minnesota, Academic Health Center, "Family Meals Promote Healthy Eating," November 9, 2004, www.ahc.umn.edu/news/releases/meals110904, accessed July 6, 2007.

10. Ibid.

11. Laurette Willis, "God's Heavenly Weigh: Garnish Your Plate with Praise," in *BASIC Steps to Godly Fitness* (Eugene, OR: Harvest House, 2005), 60-61.

12. John 6:35.

Chapter 5—Your Fitness Personality

1. See www.ThePersonalities.com for more information.

2. Information from *Personality Plus* by Florence Littauer, copyright © 1992 by Florence Littauer. Used by permission of Florence Littauer and Fleming H. Revell Company. Not to be reproduced. Copies of Personality Plus and Personality Profiles may be ordered from: CLASS, 2201 San Pedro Drive NE, Albuquerque, NM 87110 or go to www.thepersonalities.com or call 800-433-6633.

3. "The fear of man brings a snare, but whoever trusts in the LORD shall be safe" (Proverbs 29:25).

4. For stretching DVDs and books, check out material by Bob Anderson, including his book *Stretching.* Also check out Brad Walker's information at www.thestretchinghandbook.com.

5. Hebrews 6:12.

6. Isaiah 26:3.

Chapter 6—Fitness for the Busy Woman

1. 1 Timothy 4:8.

2. See 1 Corinthians 9:24-26; Galatians 2:2; 5:7; Philippians 2:16; 2 Timothy 4:7.

3. Henry J. Montoye, et al., "Measuring Physical Activity and Energy Expenditure," eds. M.E. Fowler, et al., *Human Kinetics,* (1996):97-115.

4. Romans 12:1.

5. 1 Corinthians 6:19.

6. Ephesians 6:17.

7. Galatians 6:8.

8. 1 Thessalonians 5:17.

9. John 4:24.

10. "Knowing this first, that no prophecy of Scripture is of any private interpretation" (2 Peter 1:20).

11. John 6:57-58,60.

12. John 6:63.

13. John 17:17.

14. Laurette Willis, "A Journey of 10,000 Steps Begins with One," in *BASIC Steps to Godly Fitness* (Eugene, OR: Harvest House, 2005), 98.

Chapter 7—Breathing—Escape the Shallows

1. Deuteronomy 18:9-14.

2. 1 Corinthians 9:27.

3. John 10:10.

4. 1 Corinthians 2:16.

5. Matthew 6:7.

6. Psalm 42:11.

Chapter 8—20 Minutes to Be Fit for the King

1. U.S. Department of Health and Human Services, *Physical Activity and Health: A Report of the Surgeon General,* Executive Summary (Atlanta: Centers for Disease Control and Prevention, 1996), www.cdc.gov/nccdphp/sgr/summary.htm and www.cdc.gov/nccdphp/sgr/pdf/execsumm.pdf, accessed March 14, 2007; U.S. Department of Agriculture and Department of Health and Human Services, *Dietary Guidelines for Americans* (Washington, D.C.: Government Printing Office, 2005), http://www.healthierus.gov/dietaryguidelines.

2. John M. Jakicic, et al., "Effect of Exercise Duration and Intensity on Weight Loss in Overweight, Sedentary Women," *Journal of the American Medical Association,* 290, no. 10 (September 10, 2003):1323-30; John M. Jakicic, et al., "Effects of Intermittent Exercise and Use of Home Exercise Equipment on Adherence, Weight Loss, and Fitness in Overweight Women: A Randomized Trial," *Journal of the American Medical Association,* 282 (1999):1554-60, cited in John M. Jakicic and Amy D. Otto, "Physical Activity Considerations for the Treatment and Prevention of Obesity," *American Journal of Clinical Nutrition,* 82, no. 1 (2005):226-29, www.ajcn.org/cgi/reprint/82/1/226S.pdf, accessed July 7, 2007.

3. U.S. Department of Agriculture and Department of Health and Human Services, *Dietary Guidelines for Americans* (Washington, D.C.: Government Printing Office, 2005), www.health.gov/dietaryguidelines/dga2005/document/html/chapter3. htm, accessed July 30, 2007.

4. Cris A. Slentz, et al., "Effects of the Amount of Exercise on Body Weight, Body Composition, and Measures of Central Obesity," *Archives of Internal Medicine,* 164, no. 1 (January 12, 2004):31-39, www.ncbi.nlm.nih.gov/entrez/query. fcgi?cmd=Retrieve&db=pubmed&dopt=Abstract&list_uids=14718319&query_hl=31&itool=pubmed_docsum, accessed March 14, 2007.

5. Genesis 8:22.

6. Zechariah 4:10 NLT.

7. Deuteronomy 34:7.

8. Psalm 103:1,5.

9. To learn more about Slow-Cadence Exercise, visit www.PraiseMoves.com.

Chapter 9—PraiseMoves®—The Christian Alternative to Yoga

1. Lisa Takeuchi Cullen-Mahtomedi, "Stretching for Jesus," *Time* magazine, August 29, 2005, www.time.com/time/magazine/article/0,9171,1098937,00. html, accessed March 22, 2007.

2. Quoted in Darryl E. Owens, "Bible, Yoga Strike a Pose," *Orlando Sentinel,* May 2, 2006, in Worldwide Religious News, "North America, United States, Hinduism," www.wwrn.org/article.php?idd=21366&sec=51&con=4, accessed June 30, 2007.

3. Susan Bordenkircher, *Yoga for Christians: A Christ-Centered Approach to Physical and Spiritual Health Through Yoga* (Nashville: Thomas Nelson, 2006).

4. Genesis 24:63.

5. Roger Steer, comp., *Spiritual Secrets of George Müller* (Wheaton, IL: Harold Shaw, 1985), 61-62.

Chapter 10—21 Days to Total Fitness

1. To learn more about Hebrew word pictures, I recommend the work of Dr. Frank T. Seekins at www.livingwordpictures.com or call (602)867-0903 for his teaching materials. Some of his books and CDs are also available at www.PraiseMoves.com.

2. 1 Corinthians 1:27.

3. 2 Corinthians 12:10.

4. Matthew 18:20.

5. "Whenever you stand praying, if you have anything against anyone, forgive him, that your Father in heaven may also forgive you your trespasses" (Mark 11:25).

6. "Husbands, likewise, dwell with [your wives] with understanding, giving honor to the wife, as to the weaker vessel, and as being heirs together of the grace of life, that your prayers may not be hindered" (1 Peter 3:7).

7. Zechariah 4:6.

8. William Shakespeare, "We are such stuff as dreams are made on, and our little life is rounded with a sleep," "Prospero," *The Tempest,* act 4, scene 1.

9. "We are ambassadors for Christ, as though God were pleading through us: we implore you on Christ's behalf, be reconciled to God" (2 Corinthians 5:20).

10. Hebrews 5:12-14.

11. 2 Timothy 2:21.

12. "He who has entered His rest has himself also ceased from his works as God did from His" (Hebrews 4:10).

13. "Now thanks be to God who always leads us in triumph in Christ, and through us diffuses the fragrances of His knowledge in every place" (2 Corinthians 2:14 AMP).

14. 1 Peter 5:6-7.

15. Hebrews 11:11.

16. Exodus 12:23-25.

17. 1 Peter 1:18-19.

18. Ephesians 4:27 AMP.

19. Luke 10:19.

20. Isaiah 54:17 AMP, brackets in original.

21. 1 Peter 2:9 (royal priesthood); Revelation 1:6; 5:10 (kings and priests).

22. Psalm 132:9 and Isaiah 61:10 (righteousness); Psalm 30:11 (gladness); 1 Peter 5:5 (humility).

23. 1 Chronicles 4:10.
24. Proverbs 18:16.
25. Ephesians 6:10.
26. Jeremiah 29:11.
27. 1 Kings 19:12.
28. Matthew 12:34.
29. Ephesians 4:15.
30. Psalm 141:3.
31. Psalm 19:14.
32. James 1:17 NIV.
33. Galatians 5:22-23 NLT.
34. John 3:30.
35. 2 Corinthians 4:18.
36. Exodus 34:28-30.
37. Ecclesiastes 3:11.
38. Colossians 3:23-24.

Congratulations and Keep Going!

1. Based on Philippians 4:13.

A Special Invitation

1. Acts 2:21.
2. Romans 10:9,13.

More Great Fitness Products

from Laurette Willis

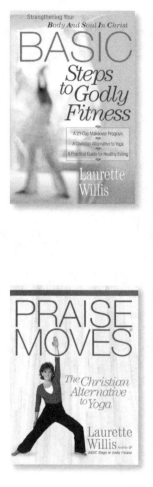

BASIC STEPS TO GODLY FITNESS

In this uniquely integrated program, certified personal trainer and aerobic instructor Laurette Willis shares her BASIC (Body And Soul In Christ), step-by-step plan so you can achieve great health in body, soul, and spirit. Convinced that diets alone don't work, Laurette shows how lasting change starts on the inside. She leads you through a process that turn mundane daily activities and exercises into acts of worship, develop a healthy self-image through forgiveness and freedom from addiction, and experience God's transforming power through praise, prayer, and fasting. You'll find plenty of practical opportunities for growth, including an introduction to PraiseMoves™, Laurette's innovative Christian system of worship and exercise that she calls "the Christian alternative to yoga."

PRAISEMOVES™ DVD

For 22 years Laurette studied yoga and endured a difficult journey through New Age beliefs. When she became a Christian, she was given the desire to create a Christian alternative to yoga. As you put the PraiseMoves principles and activities into action, you'll experience better flexibility and balance, lose weight and gain endurance, nurture a rich, meaningful prayer life, ease depression and stress and inspire joy, and develop a deep knowledge of Scripture.

This DVD provides two workouts—60 and 20 minutes—that are easy, effective, and intended for all fitness levels. You'll be uplifted and inspired as you incorporate this time of worship, health, and rejuvenation into your daily walk with God.

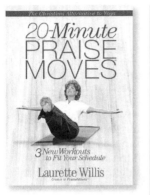

20-MINUTE PRAISEMOVES™ DVD

Are you looking for a Christ-centered alternative to Yoga for an exercise program? Laurette offers three 20-minute workouts that strengthen, tone, and increase your (beginner, intermediate, advanced) body's flexibility while renewing your mind and nourishing your spirit on God's Word. Each "posture" is linked to Scripture to transform workouts into times of worship. While reducing stress, improving circulation, and losing weight, you can energize to optional Walkin' Wisdom Warm-ups and learn God's Word through beautifully flowing Scripture sequences. *20 Minute PraiseMoves* also includes an instructional segment with exercise tips, detailed posture moves, and postures for the beginner as well as the advanced PraiseMover.

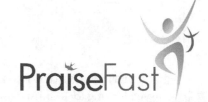

PraiseFast

A spiritual approach to lasting weight loss!

TWO REVOLUTIONARY TRUTHS COMBINED

Is there a connection between your spiritual life and how you eat? Yes! The key to weight loss is aligning your spiritual and physical needs. And the terrific news is you can find true fulfillment and satisfaction in Christ! PraiseFast uniquely combines Scripture meditation, exercise, and a dietary plan to help you lose excess weight and grow spiritually strong. And the stronger you get, the easier it is to avoid temptation and live an active, healthy lifestyle!

The PraiseFast program includes:

- *PraiseFast* (book)
- *PraiseFast Workbook*
- Delicious PraiseFast Meal Replacement shakes
- Fit Bands with 6 lbs. resistance
- Fit Bands workout sheet with Scriptures
- Daily Walk with the Lord's Prayer cards and a lanyard
- *Gimme Ten Workout* DVD and *PraiseMoves Alphabetics* DVD
- Shaker bottle
- Optional: PraiseFast Super Greens and RenewTrim Body Sculpting Formula

For more information, check out:

www.PraiseFast.com or
www.PraiseMoves.com

or call

800-211-8446